NURSING
DOCUMENTATION
HANDBOOK

D0887689

NURSING DOCUMENTATION HANDBOOK

T.M. MARRELLI, RN, MA

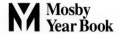

St. Louis   Baltimore   Boston   Chicago   London   Philadelphia   Sydney   Toronto

Mosby Year Book
Dedicated to Publishing Excellence

Editor: N. Darlene Como
Project Manager: Gayle May Morris
Production Editor: Judith Bange
Design: Jeanne Wolfgeher

NOTE TO THE READER: The author and publisher have diligently verified the nursing considerations discussed for accuracy and compatibility with officially accepted standards at the time of publication. With continual advancements in practice and great variety in particular patient needs, we recommend that the reader consult the latest literature and exercise professional judgment in using the guidelines in this book.

Printed in the United States of America

Mosby–Year Book Inc.
11830 Westline Industrial Drive
St. Louis, MO 63146

Library of Congress Cataloging-in-Publication Data
Marrelli, T. M.
    Nursing documentation handbook / T.M. Marrelli.
    p. cm.
    Includes bibliographical references and index.
    ISBN 0-8016-3120-3
    1. Nursing records—Handbooks, manuals, etc. I. Title.
    [DNLM: 1. Documentation—handbooks. 2. Nursing Process—handbooks.
    3. Nursing Records—handbooks. 4. Patient Care Planning—handbooks.
    WY 39 M359n]
RT50.M37 1992
610.73—dc20
DNLM/DLC
for Library of Congress   91-22827
                                                            CIP

MS/DC 9 8 7 6 5 4 3 2 1

PROFESSIONAL REVIEWERS

◆

These colleagues reviewed specific sections of the text, based on their areas of expertise. Their input ensured up-to-date information. The author and publisher thank them for their invaluable guidance.

John Blue, BS, MDiv
Department of Veteran Affairs Medical Center
Wichita, Kansas

Colleen Dantoni, RN, BSN
Shift Coordinator
Baltimore County General Hospital
Baltimore, Maryland

Jane E. Dohne, RN, BSN
University of Maryland Hospital
Progressive Care Unit
Baltimore, Maryland

Carroll Tollner Fernstrom, OTR/L
Annapolis, Maryland

Olga Makara Gordon, RNC, BS
Maternal-Child Health Instructor
Annapolis, Maryland

Neil Hartman, PT, MPH
U.S. Public Health Service
Shrewsbury, Pennsylvania

Christine Kowalski, RN
Nurse Consultant
Hallmark Healthcare
Towson, Maryland

Vicki E. Long, CNM, MSN
Annapolis OB/GYN Associates
Annapolis, Maryland

Charles Morgan, RRA, CPQA
President
Morgan and Associates
Annapolis, Maryland

Jane Ostmann, RN, MS, CCRN
Continuing Education, Critical Care
Cape Fear Valley Medical Center
Fayetteville, North Carolina

Martha Rappoli, RN
Rockport, Massachusetts

JoAnn Richardson, BSN, ET
Nurse Manager
Staffing and Nursing Information Systems
Anne Arundel Medical Center
Annapolis, Maryland

Susan Riggs, MSW
National Hospice Organization Board Member
Baltimore, Maryland

Mary Deeley Shoffeitt, RN, MS
Clinical Nurse
Woodbine, Maryland

Elizabeth K. Tanner, RN, PhD
Assistant Professor
University of Maryland School of Nursing
Baltimore, Maryland

Thomas Walsh, MD
Family Practice
Severna Park, Maryland

Linda Whitby, MD
Clinton, Maryland

PREFACE

◆

This book contains a series of documentation examples and guidelines for nurses that are easily referenced by the patient's clinical problems. As hospitals and other inpatient settings are experiencing decreasing lengths of stays and increasing patient acuity, the professional nurse must manage more responsibilities in a shortened time frame. The goal of this book is to assist the nurse in efficiently and effectively documenting patient care in the clinical record.

This book uses the nursing process to assist the nurse in achieving two objectives: meeting patient goals and simultaneously creating effective documentation. The easy-to-use format, with patient problems categorized alphabetically, will help the nurse to remember the myriad skills he or she brings to the patients bedside daily. These standards can be applied in orientation, education, and clinical case reviews, as well as at the patient's bedside. The generation of clear documentation requires a learning process. This book integrates the documentation needed for practice with actual clinical conditions.

Some special devices have been included to make this book easy to use. In the clinical material certain standard abbreviations are used throughout to simplify the written material and to allow the reader to quickly refer to needed information. If any abbreviation is unclear, check its meaning in Appendix C, Key Abbreviations. The documentation guidelines are alphabetized in all areas in Part Two on medical-surgical care, Part Three on hospice care, and Part Four on maternal child care. These areas are cross-referenced for easy access to the information. For example, care for arthritis is actually under the heading Osteoarthritis, but it is included in the table of contents as Arthritis with the page number for Osteoarthritis. For a more detailed discussion of how to use this book for care planning and other aspects of documenting patient care, see How to Use This Handbook to Streamline Documentation.

HOW TO USE THIS HANDBOOK TO STREAMLINE DOCUMENTATION

◆

Nursing entries in the clinical record are valued for the wealth of patient information they contain. It is nurses who comfort and care for patients 24 hours a day. It is nurses who coordinate all activities related to the patient. These activities are multifaced and range from clinical tests to therapeutic interventions. It is to the professional nurse that patients and their families and friends look for solace and expertise.

How does documentation relate to these important nursing responsibilities? What is the role of documentation in nursing care? Is it writing a note every shift or updating the care planning record every 24 hours? Documentation includes the all-encompassing realm of *written* communication. All other communications, verbal and nonverbal, other than written, simply appear never to have occurred. As a result, the remembering and recording of what care occurred, the patient's response, and myriad other details, take on new importance in the clinical record.

The goal of this book is to facilitate succinct documentation that assists the nurse in thoroughly documenting the care given to patients while minimizing the time required for that documentation. The initial chapters (Part One) describe the clinical record. Coverage includes the formats of clinical records, common types of nursing documentation systems, and the actual creation of effective documentation. These chapters also provide general guidelines for complete and effective documentation.

In Parts Two through Four, documentation guidelines are presented for common medical diagnoses/patient problems in medical-surgical care, hospice care, and maternal/child care. The diagnoses or patient problems are listed alphabetically. Thus when caring for a patient with diabetes mellitus and an open wound, the nurse might refer to the following clinical topics: diabetes mellitus, amputation, and wound care. The documentation guidelines provided can be used throughout the clinical record, regardless of the nursing documentation system in use at the health care facility. The format of the book's documentation guidelines can assist the busy nurse in quickly identifying interventions, data, or goals/outcomes that may be appropriate for a specific patient.

The following descriptions explain numbered entries for each clinical topic.

1. Assessment of the patient problem

This assessment is the subjective data and is often the assessment of what the patient, family, or caregiver perceives to be the problem. For SOAP notes, this is the "S." This assessment is one of the most important pieces of information that a patient provides. Obtaining this data requires good listening skills, as well as respect and empathy. The patients perception of the problem is a nursing problem needing nursing management.

2. Associated nursing diagnoses

This section includes the nursing diagnoses approved by the North American Nursing Diagnosis Association (NANDA) that are often correlated with the clinical problem. These nursing diagnoses are the identified focus for intervention by nurses and are used in the care planning record, the problem identification list, and throughout the clinical record. All or some of the diagnoses listed may be appropriate for a specific patient.

3. Examples of objective data for documentation

This section lists measurable or observable criteria specific to the clinical problem. These objective indicators are factual and can be observed. An example might be a patient crying or a temperature of 101° F rectally.

4. Examples of the assessment of the data

This section lists likely nurses' judgments based on the objective findings listed in Section 3. For example, the temperature of 101° F indicates that the patient is febrile, and, based on this assessment, the nurse has information on which to base the next care decision.

5. Examples of potential medical problems for this patient

This section enumerates some of the pathological conditions that may occur as either part of the progression of the disease or a side effect of treatment, or for other reasons. An example might be a fat embolism after bony trauma or a urinary tract infection in a patient with an indwelling urinary catheter.

6. Examples of the documentation of potential nursing interventions/actions

Nursing interventions or actions that may be appropriate for the patient are specified in this section. NOTE: The physician order(s) should always be checked prior to performing any intervention. Some, none, or all of the interventions/actions listed may be appropriate and must be individualized for a specific patient.

7. Examples of the evaluations of the interventions/actions

The evaluations listed in this section are the responses or outcomes of the interventions or implemented plans. For example, if the intervention is the administration of an antiemetic medication, the evaluation might be that the patient ceased vomiting or verbalized relief from nausea. The evaluation may be positive or negative, or there may be no change identified. There should be an evaluation statement for every nursing intervention.

8. Other services that may be indicated and their associated interventions and goals/outcomes

This section focuses on interdisciplinary patient care. For example, the patient who has suffered a cerebrovascular accident often needs rehabilitation services such as physical therapy (PT), occupational therapy (OT), and speech- language pathology (SLP) services.

The services listed by discipline are not meant to be exclusive and/or all-inclusive for any diagnosis. Because this book is written primarily for nurses, the nursing interventions/actions are more extensive. However, this is not to say that other disciplines (e.g., PT, OT, chaplaincy, or SLP services) might not also address the same or similar interventions and goals. For example, respiratory therapists perform chest percussion, as do nurses and physical therapists. In addition, speech-language pathologists do swallowing evaluations at some hospitals whereas at others occupational therapists do the swallowing assessments. Our desire to create a concise, quick reference handbook precluded providing detailed listings of interventions for disciplines other than nursing. This is not meant in any way to diminish the importance or value of all of the variously skilled personnel whose services are needed by patients. On the contrary, the intent of this book is to encourage an interdisciplinary approach to patient care.

9. Nursing goals and outcomes.

These nursing goals and/or outcomes listed in this section are based on the patient's diagnoses or problem(s). They are objective and measurable goals that may be accomplished by nursing care, and they may be used in the patient care planning record, throughout the charting method the hospital uses, and in narrative entries. These guidelines will assist in the determination of goal achievement and in evaluating discharge planning processes. Usually, where stated goals have been reached and documented, discharge is imminent.

10. Potential discharge plans for this patient.

The discharge plans listed in this section are the most common plans, based on the patient's diagnoses and problem(s). Clearly, these plans are specific to the patient's unique clinical course, prognoses, and wishes. They are listed to identify options that may be appropriate for a patient.

To enhance the handbook's usefulness as a quick reference and to facilitate efficient and consistent documentation, three appendixes have been included that provide information the nurse may need to refer to frequently. Appendix A lists all the NANDA-approved diagnoses using the latest NANDA terminology. Appendix B described services commonly provided by other disciplines. Appendix C lists key abbreviations to promote consistent, comprehensible documentation.

CONTENTS

PART ONE The Principles of
Documentation

PART TWO Medical-Surgical Care
Documentation Guidelines

PART THREE Hospice Care Documentation Guidelines

PART FOUR Maternal/Child Care Documentation Guidelines

APPENDIXES

BIBLIOGRAPHY, 289

PART ONE

THE PRINCIPLES OF DOCUMENTATION

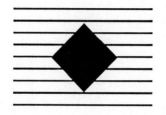

CHAPTER 1

Documentation: An Overview

◆

Nurses and nursing practice are described every day to those who read a medical record. Nursing entries that appear in that record reflect the standard of nursing care, as well as the particular care given to a specific patient. Other health team members make decisions for care based on nursing notes. And today, numerous third parties make legal and quality judgments, as well as administrative and reimbursement decisions, and perform other actions peripheral to the actual care of the patient based on the medical record.

Nurses have many varied responsibilities, all ultimately directed toward patient care. Because of this, the actual task of documentation must sometimes be relegated to harried moments toward the end of the shift. However, the definition of the word *documentation* provides information on documentation's important role. *Webster's New World Dictionary* defines documentation as "the supplying of documentary evidence. . . and the collecting, abstracting, and coding of printed or written information for future reference." This simple definition fits all the varied roles that documentation, or the process of documenting and demonstrating delivery of patient care, assumes in health care.

Today, the typical medical record may be viewed by a minimum of 10 persons during the patient's initial 24 hours in the health care facility. These persons may include the attending or admitting physician, three nurses on different shifts, a utilization review specialist, several nurse aides, and a dietitian. They may also include a surgeon, an anesthesiologist, and various technicians and therapists. With so many persons depending on the medical record as a reliable source of information on a patient, the importance of the documentation contained in the record becomes evident.

The professional nurse's entries in the patient's clinical record are recognized as a significant contribution that documents the standard of care provided to a patient. As the practice of nursing has become more complex, so, too, have the factors that influence the roles of documentation. These factors include requirements of regulatory agencies, health insurance payors, accreditation organizations, consumers of health care, and legal entities. The nurse must try to satisfy these various requirements all at once, often with precious few moments in which to accomplish this important task.

Any nurse writing a clinical entry today could be striving to simultaneously meet the standards of the Joint Commission on Accreditation of Healthcare Organizations, various health insurers, state and federal laws and regulations, and other professional organizations. Fortunately, most hospitals have integrated many of these requirements, where possible, into hospital policy and/or procedure manuals. The documentation-related standards of the Joint Commission on Accreditation of Health Care Organizations and the American Nurses' Association influence nursing documentation in most settings; thus they have been included in this book for your reference (see Chapters 4 and 5.)

The clinical record written today is also the nurse's best defense against any litigation where malpractice or negligence is alleged.

The increased specialization of health care

providers and the complexity of patient problems and associated technology have contributed to multiple and varied services being provided to patients. The medical record is the only source of written communication, and sometimes the only source of any communication, for all team members. The members not only contribute their individual assessments of interventions and outcomes, but actually base their subsequent actions on the record of events provided by another team member. This record is the only document that chronicles a patient's stay from admission through discharge. As such, the actual entries must be recorded as soon as possible after a change in the patient's condition is noted, an intervention is provided, or the response to a treatment is observed.

There are five major factors that contribute to the increased emphasis on nursing documentation.

1. The current economics of our health care system and utilization management

In response to spiraling health care costs, third-party payors (government, commercial, and business self-insurers) have increased their scrutiny and control of hospital resources. Such programs, called utilization review or utilization management, have been influential in decreasing hospital lengths of stays. Thus patient populations who would have required an extended hospital stay 5 to 10 years ago now experience much briefer hospitalizations. In addition, many surgeries and other procedures today are provided on an outpatient-only basis.

In general, decreased lengths of stays increase patients' nursing care needs during the shortened time period. The phrase often heard to describe this phenomenon is "quicker and sicker."

The clinical record is the source by which third-party payors make payment or denial decisions. It is nursing documentation that often becomes the basis for that payment decision.

2. The emphasis on quality assurance/quality assessment in health care

As hospital quality assurance programs have evolved, patient outcomes are recognized as valid indicators of quality of care. Clinical documentation becomes the written record demonstrating the nursing process and movement toward achieving patient goals and positive outcomes.

The new interdisciplinary focus of quality assurance efforts creates an atmosphere for the entire health team to work together to achieve patient outcomes. The clinical documentation is the written evidence of this collaboration in the format of team meetings, conferences, or other activity.

3. The emphasis on standardization of care, and policies and procedures

All patients are entitled to a certain level or standard of nursing care. As patients become more proactive consumers in their purchase of health services care, patient satisfaction with the care provided becomes the key to a hospital's reputation and ultimate survival. Nurses, because of their healing skills and other areas of proficiency, are pivotal to fostering patient satisfaction. It is also known that generally satisfied patients are less likely to sue. The role of the nurse as patient advocate, listener, and teacher has become widely accepted in recent years.

4. The furthering recognition and empowering of the nursing profession

Although there are more nurses in the work force

than ever before, there continues to be a need for qualified professional nurses. The nurse's notes can become the factor by which documented quality (or negligence) becomes demonstrated quality (or negligence). All health care professions, including nursing, have recognized standards of care. As society has become more litigious, the nurse must be aware of state nurse practice acts and other accepted standards of care. These standards of care are the *minimum* level that any patient can expect in similar circumstances. Other standards include local hospital policy and procedures, state or federal regulations, and the published standards of the professional nursing organizations.[1] This is the reason for the necessity of keeping current and informed of the standards of professional nursing practice through affiliation with nursing specialty groups or other professional groups.

Some examples of hospitals' nursing standards of care are:

- Every patient shall have a nursing assessment that is comprehensive, addresses specific patient needs, is performed by a registered nurse at least every_____hours, and is documented in the clinical record.
- Every patient shall have a written plan of care that is developed and revised by a registered nurse, and is updated every_____ hours or more frequently based on the patient's condition.
- Discharge planning will begin on admission, will include collaboration with other members of the health care team, and will involve the patient, family, and caregiver(s).

Through complete and effective documentation, nursing demonstrates that the standard of care has been met.

5. The emphasis on effectiveness and efficiency in health care

As hospitals continue to streamline their operations, administrative tasks done historically by nurses are being reconsidered. Repetition or duplication of documentation has been an area of appropriate concern to both the nurse and management. Many health care facilities have moved toward recording things only once in the record. Quality, not quantity, is now emphasized with regard to documentation.

All of these factors have created an environment in which the nurse has increased responsibilities to be undertaken in a shortened time period because of decreased patient lengths of stays. The medical record becomes the only written account of these briefer stays. Chapter 2 further examines the important role of the medical record.

REFERENCE

1. Guide GW: *Legal issues in nursing: a source book for practice,* Norwalk, Conn, 1985, Appleton & Lange.

CHAPTER 2

The Medical Record

◆

The functions of documentation in the medical record relate to the facts that this record is:

- The only written source that chronicles a patient's stay
- The primary source for reference and communication among the members of the health care team
- The only text that supports insurance coverage and/or denial
- The only evidence of the basis on which patient care decisions were made
- The only legal record
- The primary foundation for the evaluation of the care provided
- The basis for staff education or other study
- The objective source for the hospital's licensing and accreditation review (e.g., the Joint Commission on Accreditation of Health Care Organizations, the American Osteopathic Association Standards)

Various entities are interested in different aspects of clinical documentation. The following is an example. Mr. Smith is admitted to the community hospital for a hip fracture repair. In the comprehensive assessment, done on admission, the prudent nurse identifies potential problems. This includes information from Mr. Smith's daughter, his caregiver, that whenever he is away from home he becomes confused, agitated, and forgetful. One night, 5 days postoperatively, Mr. Smith is found on the floor.

Who is interested in Mr. Smith's chart, and why?

- Mr. Smith's surgeon, physical therapists, and others who have been planning his care and working on his level of mobility to achieve his prehospitalization level of functioning
- The hospital risk manager to evaluate the incident and plan for possible outcomes
- The quality assurance and nursing departments, which are studying and tracking falls to recommend policy and/or procedure changes to decrease falls and their consequences
- The third-party payor(s) who will be concerned with the additional patient costs and days of care needed
- The licensing and accreditation body, should the chart be reviewed, to determine whether accepted standards of care were delivered; also, to determine whether nursing and administrative policies and procedures were followed
- Mr. Smith's daughter, who demands to read her father's record to find out what happened (Most hospitals have a structured process permitting such review.)
- Mr. and Mrs. Smith's attorney, should they choose to pursue litigation for alleged negligence or malpractice
- The hospital's attorney to (hopefully) show the nurse's clear documentation as the best defense demonstrating that nursing practice met accepted standards of care[1]

In this example it is hoped that the nursing documentation identified this patient to be at risk for confusion and that extra steps were taken to reduce his risk. Examples of steps taken for this patient might be that side rails were up, the patient was checked at q___ intervals, a sitter was obtained to stay at the bedside, and the patient was relocated closer to the nursing station. All of these steps may show that extra care was taken to protect this patient. This demonstrates the role of the medical record in its function of meeting many needs, including legal, fiscal, clinical, and regulatory requirements.[2]

Because nurses must meet these myriad needs simultaneously, they should be appropriately concerned about their ability to do so. Nurses in practice today can meet these needs and produce clear and effective documentation. The following points can assist in this process:

REMEMBER

- Write legibly or print neatly. The record must be readable.

- Use permanent ink, (Appropriate ink color may depend on hospital policy.)

- For every entry, identify the time and date; sign the entry and list your title.

- Describe care provided and the patient's response to care.

- Write objectively in describing findings (e.g., behaviors).

- Write entries in consecutive and chronological order with no skipped lines or gaps.

- Write entries as soon as possible after care is provided.

- Be factual and specific.

- Use patient (or family or caregiver) quotes.

- Use the patient's name (e.g., Mr. "Smith")
- Document patient complaints or needs and their resolution.
- Be complete, accurate, and thorough.
- Write out what you are saying (avoid potentially confusing abbreviations).
- Chart only care you provided.
- Promptly document a change in the patient's condition and the actions taken based on that change.
- Write the patient's, family's, or caregiver's response to teaching.
- To correct an error: (1) draw a single line through the erroneous entry, (2) briefly describe the error (e.g., wrong date, chart), and (3) add your signature, the date, and the time.

AVOID

- Relying on memory
- Whiting out or erasing entries. (Such changes may appear to be an attempt to cover up incriminating entries.)
- Crossing out words beyond recognition
- Making assumptions, drawing conclusions, or blaming
- Leaving blank spaces between entries and your signature
- Recording late entries
- Leaving gaps in documentation
- Using abbreviations except where they are clear

and appear on the hospital's list of acceptable abbreviations.

CHECKLIST FOR DOCUMENTATION

- Try to look at the documentation objectively; does it tell the story of the patient's progress (or lack of progress) and the interventions implemented based on your evaluation?

- Are telephone calls and other communications with physicians or other team members documented? Do they explain what happened, what actions were then ordered and carried out, and the patient's response to the orders?

- Is use of the nursing process demonstrated? Look for the nursing diagnoses, the written assessment, evidence of care planning, implementation of the interventions and actions, and assessment of the patient's response and further evaluation?

- Are there frequent entries that show care provided?

- Is there documentation of goal achievement and/or progress toward goals and outcomes? Are the goals realistic, measurable, and clear to other readers?

- If progress has not occurred as planned, are the reasons for this clearly stated?

- Is the patient's response to each patient care intervention/action described? For example, for parenteral drug administration is the specific site of administration, the patient's position, and the drug's dosage, actions, and response documented?

- Are the interventions modified, based on the

patient's response, where appropriate?

- Is there written communication among multidisciplinary team members regarding patient goals/outcomes? For example, is there documentation of a discharge planning conference?

- Does the charting show continuity of care and further coordination based on the entries?

- The clinical record entries represent the nurse and the standards of care provided. Do they reflect current professional standards? Are they neat and legible? (Remember, legibility is a standard.)

- Is there documentation of the patient's activities of daily living (ADL) status? For example, "Patient has used guad cane to assist ambulation for 2 years."

- Generally, does the documentation tell the story of the patient's stay at the hospital?

- Does it make sense, or are there gaps without explanations? Are the actions of team members directed toward the same goals?

- Do the actions documented seem to contribute to the patient's receiving care that will assist in meeting the stated goals/outcomes?

- Are actions focused toward identified discharge goals/outcomes?

- Finally, do the entries reflect nursing care of the level expected by today's consumer?

Nursing documentation represents the quality of care provided. Unfortunately, if it is not written, the assumption can be made that it did not happen.

Through complete documentation, the nurse can claim credit for meeting responsibilities inherent in the profession. Documentation is a vital adjunct to providing patient care. It is the sole written record of a patient's stay and, as such, represents the care provided. Nurses can have their practice represented well through thorough, effective documentation.

REFERENCES

1. Legally speaking: careful charting—your best defense, *RN*, p 77, November 1990.
2. Glondys BA: *Today's challenge: content of the health record; documentation requirements in the medical record*, ed 2, Chicago, 1988, American Medical Record Association.

CHAPTER 3

Systems of Nursing Documentation

◆

Every hospital has its own method or standard format for nursing documentation in the clinical record. Some hospitals have designated nursing notes, and others have one area, usually interdisciplinary progress notes, where all team members, including nurses, document care. Charting has historically been viewed as being secondary to patient care. This unfortunate outlook does not reflect the value placed on the nursing entries made in the medical record. All nursing notes, regardless of type of location in the record, are nursing documentation. Whatever kind of documentation system is used, the documentation must communicate the patient's status, the specific care provided, and the response to that care. Below are brief descriptions of some of these methods and their unique characteristics.

1. **Problem-oriented medical record (POMR or POR)**

This system is best known for the order in which information is organized: the SOAP note. Dr. Weed introduced this system of documentation to be used by all who make entries into the clinical record. This method organizes information by the patient's problem. In its classic format the POMR is composed of the database, a numbered problem list, and the SOAP notes identified by the original problem list. The SOAP format has also evolved into the SOAPE,

SOAPIE, and SOAPIER notes in practice. These names are acronyms representing subjective data or information(S), objective data or information *(O)*, assessmemt *(A)*, and plan (of care) *(P)*.[1] Some institutions also use intervention *(I)*, evaluation *(E)*, and/or response *(R)*. Many modified approaches to this system are in use today.

2. Focus charting

This format was introduced in the early 1980s. As its name implies, focus charting can streamline the documentation process. This method offers an alternative way of documenting that requires less time than other methods by most standards. The format, like SOAP, has three letters that summarize the structure: DAR. These letters represent data *(D)*, action(s) *(A)*, and response(s) *(R)*. The first entry, which is placed in the left column, is the note's "focus." This can be a symptom, a problem, or the nursing diagnosis. The notes, addressing the three key components, DAR, are written to the right of the identified problem.[2]

3. Charting by exception

As the words *charting by exception* imply, only significant or abnormal findings, or exceptions to standardized, expected norms are written in the narrative notes using this method. This change in emphasis decreases the time spent documenting normal findings. Although there are differences in the application of this method at various facilities, it has several key characteristics: the integration of standardized care plans, the use of flow sheets, and the placement of some portion of the clinical record at the patient's bedside. Some hospitals have also incorporated walking rounds at change of shift so that the incoming nurse can, at a glance, see the patient and the documentation flow sheets. This method, which has been used in practice since the mid 1980s, was developed in response to the economic climate that emphasized quality care in a cost-contained environment. It standardizes assessments and other clinical findings, and has been reported to decrease repetitive entries, especially in such areas as intake and output and other flow sheets. To be successfully implemented, this system must be based on accepted standards or norms. These standards must be clear and specific to adequately define the exceptions on which this method is based.

4. Computerized documentation

Computerized nursing documentation is becoming more common in hospitals as applications for automation in nursing have increased. In some systems the nurse can select those actions or findings appropriate to a specific patient to facilitate making an entry in the clinical record. Placing a computer at the patient's bedside assists in ensuring frequent entries. In most nursing systems, however, the video display terminal (VDT) is placed in the nursing station to tie into other departments. Computerizing the record and the nursing notes may ultimately save hospitals money and increase the quality of care. Studies have shown that nursing costs can account for 30% to 40% of a hospital's operational budget. It has been estimated that the average nurse spends 2 or 3 hours per shift on administrative tasks.[3]

Nursing computer systems today are integrating the different components of the charge. For example, once the assessment is completed, an individualized care plan is developed, and from that point a patient-specific flow sheet can be generated, thus decreasing the time required for the documentation process by 40% to 50% per patient per shift. Kardexes and other components can also be generated via the computer system. Computerizing nursing documentation may decrease time spent on repetitive administrative tasks, thus allowing professional nurses to spend more time caring for patients. Maintaining the confidentiality of computerized entries without restricting legitimate retrieval of needed information is an issue that is currently being addressed by both users and system developers.

5. Narrative charting

Although there are numerous newer systems of nursing documentation, such as those described above, the narrative note continues to be predominant method for making clinical entries in the medical record.[4] Narrative charting is identified historically by lengthy entries into the record. However, all nursing documentation systems incorporate some narrative documentation. A common example is a particularly lengthy SOAPIE note that requires significant detail to communicate clinical actions and the patient's response to the nursing interventions.

◆ ◆ ◆

Many hospitals use a modified version of one or more of the documentation systems described above. The goal for all is complete documentation. In addition, regardless of the approach chosen at any hospital for nursing documentation, some key focal points remain the same. For example, the O for objective in the SOAP format is equivalent to the D for data in the focus charting method, and defined, standardized abnormal findings would be the objective data when the method of charting by exception is used. All of these methods lend themselves to the effective use of nursing diagnosis.

Chapter 4 presents the 1991 Nursing Care and Medical Record Services Standards related to documentation from the Joint Commission on Accreditation of Healthcare Organizations. The American Nurses' Association Standard I is presented in Chapter 5. The integration of this material into daily clinical documentation will assist in meeting standards of care.

REFERENCES

1. Rutkowski B: How D.R.G.s are changing your charting, *Nursing 85*, p 49, October 1985.

2. Iyer PW: New trends in charting, *Nursing 91* p 48, January 1991.

3. Carter K: Computer technology advances will help hospitals to compete, *Health* p 90, November 22.

4. Eggland ET: Charting: how and why to document your care daily—and fully, *Nursing 88*, p 76, November 1988.

CHAPTER 4

The Joint Commission on Accreditation of Healthcare Organizations' Standards Related to Documentation

NURSING CARE (NC)

Patients receive nursing care* in various settings throughout the hospital. For example, nursing care is provided in medical-surgical nursing care units, in alcohol and other drug dependence programs, in mental health nursing care units, in biopsychosocial and physical rehabilitation programs, in hospital-sponsored ambulatory clinics and services, in emergency services, in intensive care and other special care units, and in units in which surgical and other invasive procedures are performed. The standards in this chapter apply to all settings in which nursing care is provided in the hospital.

---

*As defined in relevant state, commonwealth, or territory nurse practice acts and other applicable laws and regulations, and as permitted by the hospital in accordance with these definitions. Anesthesia or obstetrical care, for example, when provided by nurses in expanded practice roles, is not defined as "nursing care."

Standard

NC.1   Patients receive nursing care based on a documented assessment of their needs.*

Required characteristics

NC.1.1   Each patient's need for nursing care related to his/her admission is assessed by a registered nurse.*

> NC.1.1.1 The assessment is conducted either at the time of admission or within a time frame preceding or following admission that is specified in hospital policy.*
>
> NC.1.1.2 Aspects of data collection may be delegated by the registered nurse.
>
> NC1.1.3 Needs are reassessed when warranted by the patient's condition.*

NC.1.2   Each patient's assessment includes consideration of biophysical, psychosocial, environmental, self-care, educational, and discharge planning factors.†

> NC.1.2.1 When appropriate, data from the patient's significant other(s) are included in the assessment.

NC.1.3   Each patient's nursing care is based on identified nursing diagnoses and/or patient care needs and patient care standards, and is consistent with the therapies of other disciplines.*

---

*The asterisked items are key factors in the accreditation decision process.

NC.1.3.1 The patient and/or significant other(s) are involved in the patient's care, as appropriate.

NC.1.3.2 Nursing staff members collaborate, as appropriate, with physicians and other clinical disciplines in making decisions regarding each patient's need for nursing care.

NC.1.3.3 Throughout the patient's stay, the patient and, as appropriate, his/her significant other(s) receive education specific to the patient's health care needs.*

NC.1.3.3.1 In preparation for discharge, continuing care needs are assessed and referrals for such care are documented in the patient's medical record.

NC.1.3.4 The patient's medical record includes documentation of*

NC.1.3.4.1 the initial assessments and reassessments;

NC.1.3.4.2 the nursing diagnoses and/or patient care needs;

NC.1.3.4.3 the interventions identified to meet the patient's nursing care needs;

NC.1.3.4.4 the nursing care provided;

NC.1.3.4.5 the patient's response to, and the outcomes of, the care provided; and

NC.1.3.4.6 the abilities of the patient and/or, as appropriate, his/her significant other(s) to manage continuing care needs after discharge.

---

*The asterisked items are key factors in the accreditation decision process.

NC.1.3.5 Nursing care data related to patient assessments, the nursing care planned, nursing interventions, and patient outcomes are permanently integrated into the clinical information system (for example, the medical record).*

NC.1.3.5.1 Nursing care data can be identified and retrieved from the clinical information system.

MEDICAL RECORD SERVICES (MR)

Standard

MR.1   The hospital maintains medical records that are documented accurately and in a timely manner, are readily accessible, and permit prompt retrieval of information, including statistical data.*

Required characteristics

MR.1.1   An adequate medical record is maintained for each individual who is evaluated or treated as an inpatient, ambulatory care patient, or emergency patient, or who receives patient care services in a hospital-administered home care program.*

MR.1.2   The purposes of the medical record are as follows:

MR.1.2.1 To serve as a basis for planning

---

*The asterisked items are key factors in the accreditation decision process.

patient care and for continuity in the evaluation of the patient's condition and treatment;

MR.1.2.2 To furnish documentary evidence of the course of the patient's medical evaluation, treatment, and change in condition during the hospital stay, during an ambulatory care or emergency visit to the hospital, or while being followed in a hospital-administered home care program;

MR.1.2.3 To document communication between the practitioner responsible for the patient and any other health care professional who contributes to the patient's care;

MR.1.2.4 To assist in protecting the legal interest of the patient, the hospital, and the practitioner responsible for the patient; and

MR.1.2.5 To provide data for use in continuing education and in research.

MR.1.3 All significant clinical information pertaining to a patient is incorporated in the patient's medical record.*

MR.1.4 The content of the medical record is sufficiently detailed and organized to enable

MR.1.4.1 the practitioner responsible for the patient to provide continuing care to

---

*The asterisked items are key factors in the accreditation decision process.

the patient, determine later what the patient's condition was at a specific time, and review the diagnostic and therapeutic procedures performed and the patient's response to treatment.*

MR.1.4.2 a consultant to render an opinion after an examination of the patient and a review of the medical record*;

MR.1.4.3 another practitioner to assume the care of the patient at any time*; and

MR.1.4.4 the retrieval of pertinent information required for utilization review and quality assurance activities.*

MR.1.5 To assure that the maximum possible information about a patient is available to the professional staff providing care, the unit record system is used.

MR.1.5.1 When it is not feasible to combine all inpatient, ambulatory care, and emergency records of an individual patient into a single unit record, a system is established to routinely assemble all divergently located record components when a patient is admitted to the hospital or appears for a prescheduled ambulatory care appointment; alternatively, there is a system that required placing, in the ambulatory care or combined ambulatory care/emergency record file, copies of pertinent portions of each inpatient medical record, such as the discharge resume, the operative note, and the pathology report.

---

*The asterisked items are key factors in the accreditation decision process.

MR.1.6 Pertinent medical information obtained on request from outside sources is filed with, but not necessarily as part of, the patient's medical record.

MR.1.6.1 Such information is available to professional staff concerned with the care and treatment of the patient.

MR.1.7 In the interest of facilitating the use of the medical record by all those authorized to review or make entries in it, as well as facilitating the retrieval of information for administrative, statistical, and quality assurance activities, it is recommended that a standardized format be developed for hospital wide use.

MR.1.7.1 The format is approved by the medical staff through its designated mechanism.

MR.1.7.2 The use of a standardized format does not preclude making improvements in the medical record that will simplify the timely recording, review, or retrieval of information while not sacrificing the required content.

MR.1.7.3 Refer also the "Quality Assurance" chapter of this *Manual*.

Standard

MR.2 The medical record contains sufficient information to identify the patient, support the diagnosis, justify the treatment, and document the course and results accurately.*

*The asterisked items are key factors in the accreditation decision process.

28

Required characteristics

MR.2.1 Although the format and forms in use in the medical record will vary, all medical records contain the following:

MR.2.1.1 Identification data.

MR.2.1.1.1 When identification data are not obtainable, the reason is entered in the record.

MR.2.1.2 The medical history of the patient.*

MR.2.1.3 As appropriate to the age of the patient, a summary of the patient's psychosocial needs.*

MR.2.1.4 Reports of relevant physical examination.*

MR.2.1.5 Diagnostic and therapeutic orders.*

MR.2.1.6 Evidence of appropriate informed consent.

MR.2.1.6.1 When consent is not obtainable, the reason is entered in the recorded.

MR.2.1.7 Clinical observations, including the results of therapy.*

MR.2.1.8 Reports of procedures, tests, and their results.*

MR.2.1.9 Conclusions at termination of hospitalization or evaluation/treatment.*

MR.2.2 Inpatient medical records include at least the following*:

*The asterisked items are key factors in the accreditation decision process.

MR.2.2.1 Identification data.

MR.2.2.1.1 These data include the patient's name, address, date of birth, and next of kin.

MR.2.2.1.2 There also is a number that identifies the patient and the patient's medical record(s).

MR.2.2.2 The medical history of the patient.*

MR.2.2.2.1 The history includes the following information:

MR.2.2.2.1.1 The chief complaint;

MR.2.2.2.1.2 Details of the present illness, including, when appropriate, assessment of the patient's emotional, behavioral, and social status;

MR.2.2.2.1.3 Relevant past, social, and family histories, appropriate to the age of the patient; and

MR.2.2.2.1.4 An inventory by body systems.

MR.2.2.2.2 Whenever possible, the medical history is obtained from the patient.

MR.2.2.2.3 In services for children and adolescents,*

MR.2.2.2.3.1 an evaluation of the patient's developmental age;

MR.2.2.2.3.2 consideration of eduational needs and daily activities, as priate;

---

*The asterisked items are key factors in the accreditation decision process.

MR.2.2.2.3.3 the parent's report or other documentation of the patient's immunization status; and

MR.2.2.2.3.4 the family's and/or guardian's expectations for, and involvement in, the assessment, treatment, and continuous care of the patient.

MR.2.2.2.4 Opinions of the interviewer are not ordinarily recorded in the body of the history.

MR.2.2.2.5 The medical history is completed within the first 24 hours of admission to inpatient services.*

MR.2.2.2.5.1 If a complete history has been obtained within a week prior to admission, such as in the office of a physician staff member or, when appropriate, the office of a qualified oral surgeon staff member (refer to the "Medical Staff" chapter, Standard MS.4, required Characteristic MS.4.3.3.1), a durable, legible copy of this report may be used in the patient's hospital medical record, provided there have been no subsequent changes or the changes have been recorded at the time of admission.

MR.2.2.2.6 Obstetric records include all prenatal information

MR.2.2.2.6.1 A durable, legible original or reproduction of the office or clinic prenatal record is acceptable.

MR.2.2.3 The report of the physical examination.*

MR.2.2.3.1 The report reflects a comprehensive current physical assessment.*

MR.2.2.3.2 The physical assessment is completed within the first 24 hours of admission to inpatient services.*

MR.2.2.3.2.1 If a complete physical examination has been performed within a week prior to admission, such as in the office of a physician staff member or, when appropriate, the office of a qualified oral surgeon staff member (refer to "Medical Staff" chapter, Standard MS.4, Required Characteristic MS.4.3.3.1), a durable, legible copy of this report may be used in the patient's hospital medical record, provided there have been no changes subsequent to the original examination or the changes have been recorded at the time of admission.

MR.2.2.3.3 The recorded physical examination is authenticated by a physician or, when appropriate, by a qualified oral surgeon member of the medical staff.

MR.2.2.3.4 When a patient is readmitted within 30 days for the same or a related problem, an interval history and physical examination reflecting any sub-

*The asterisked items are key factors in the accreditation decision process.

sequent changes may be used in the medical record, provided the original information is readily available, such as in a unit record.

MR.2.2.3.5 The medical record documents a current, thorough physical examination prior to the performance of surgery.*

MR.2.2.4 A statement of the conclusions or impressions drawn from the admission history and physical examination.*

MR.2.2.5 A statement of the course of action planned for the patient while in the hospital.*

MR.2.2.5.1 There is a periodic review of the planned course of action, as appropriate.

MR.2.2.6 Diagnostic and therapeutic orders.*

MR.2.2.6.1 Such orders include those written by medical staff members, by physicians in training status, and by other individuals within the authority of their clinical privileges.

MR.2.2.6.2 Verbal orders of authorized individuals are accepted and transcribed by qualified personnel who are identified by title or category in the medical staff rules and regulations.

MR.2.2.6.3 The medical staff defines any category of diagnostic or therapeutic verbal orders associated with any potential hazard to the patient.

_____

*The asterisked items are key factors in the accreditation decision process.

MR.2.2.6.3.1 Such orders are authenticated within 24 hours by the practitioner responsible for the patient.

MR.2.2.7 Evidence of appropriate informed consent.

MR.2.2.7.1 A policy on informed consent is developed by the medical staff and governing body and is consistent with any legal requirements.

MR.2.2.7.2 The medical record contains evidence of informed consent for procedures and treatments for which it is required by the policy on informed consent.

MR.2.2.8 Clinical observations.*

MR.2.2.9 Progress notes made by the medical staff.*

MR.2.2.9.1 Progress notes give a pertinent chronological report of the patient's course in the hospital and reflect any change in condition and the results of treatment.

MR.2.2.9.2 Pertinent progress notes are also made by individuals so authorized by the medical staff, such as house staff members and individuals who have been granted clinical privileges.

MR.2.2.10 Consultation reports.*

MR.2.2.10.1 Each consultation report contains a written opinion by the

---

*The asterisked items are key factors in the accreditation decision process.

consultant that reflects, when appropriate, an actual examination of the patient and the patient's medical record(s).

MR.2.2.11 Nursing notes and entries by nonphysicians that contain pertinent, meaningful observations and information.*

MR.2.2.11.1 When oxygen is prescribed for newborn infants, its use is recorded at least as an oxygen concentration percentage and at regular, defined intervals, in accordance with a written policy of the newborn nursery.

MR.2.2.11.2 Opinions requiring medical judgment are written or authenticated only by medical staff members, house staff members, and other individuals who have been granted clinical privileges.

MR.2.2.12 Reports of procedures, tests, and their results.*

MR.2.2.12.1 All diagnostic and therapeutic procedures are recorded and authenticated in the medical record.

MR.2.2.12.1.1 Any reports from organizations outside the hospital may also be included, in which case the source organization is identified in the report.

MR.2.2.12.2 The individual who is responsible for the patient authenticates and records a preoperative diagnosis prior to surgery.

_____

*The asterisked items are key factors in the accreditation decision process.

MR.2.2.12.3 Operative reports are dictated or written in the medical record immediately after surgery and contain a description of the findings, the technical procedures used, the specimens removed, the postoperative diagnosis, and the name of the primary surgeon and any assistants.*

MR.2.2.12.3.1 The completed operative report is authenticated by the surgeon and filed in the medical record as soon as possible after surgery.

MR.2.2.12.3.2 When there is a transcription and/or filing delay, a comprehensive operative progress note is entered in the medical record immediately after surgery to provide pertinent information for use by any individual who is required to attend to the patient.

MR.2.2.13 Reports of pathology and clinical laboratory examination, radiology and nuclear medicine examinations or treatment, anesthesia records, and any other diagnostic or therapeutic procedures.*

MR.2.2.13.1 Such reports are completed promptly and are filed in the record within 24 hours of completion, if possible.

MR.2.2.14 Medical records of donors and recipients of transplants.

---

*The asterisked items are key factors in the accreditation decision process.

MR.2.2.14.1 When an organ or tissue is obtained from a living donor for transplantation purposes, the medical records of the donor and recipient fulfill the requirements for any surgical inpatient medical record.

MR.2.2.14.2 When a donor organ or tissue is obtained from a decreased patient, the medical record of the donor includes the data and time of death, documentation by and identification of the physician who determined the death, and documentation of the removal of the organ or tissue.

MR.2.2.14.3 When a cadaveric organ or cadaveric tissue is removed for purposes of donation, the removal is documented in the donor's medical record.

MR.2.2.14.4 Reference should be made to pertinent state laws for other medical record requirements.

MR.2.2.15 Conclusions at termination of hospitalization.*

MR.2.2.15.1 Conclusions include the provisional diagnosis or reasons(s) for admission, the principal and additional or associated diagnosis, the clinical resume or final progress note, and, when appropriate, the autopsy report.

MR.2.2.15.2 All relevant diagnoses established by the time of discharge, as well as all operative procedures preformed, are recorded, using acceptable disease and operative terminology that includes topography and etiology, as appropriate.

MR.2.2.15.3 The clinical resume concisely recapitulates the reason for hospitalization, the significant findings, the procedures performed and treatment rendered, the condition of the patient on discharge, and any specific instructions given to the patient and/or family, as pertinent.*

MR.2.2.15.3.1 Consideration is given to instructions relating to physical activity, medication, diet, and follow-up care.*

MR.2.2.15.4 The condition of the patient on discharge is stated in terms that permit a specific measurable comparison with the condition on admission, avoiding the use of vague relative terminology, such as "improved."

MR.2.2.15.5 When preprinted instructions are given to the patient or family, the record so indicates and a sample of the instruction sheet in use at the time is on file in the medical record department.

MR.2.2.15.6 If authorized in writing by the patient or his legally qualified representative, a copy of the clinical resume is sent to any known medical practitioner and/or medical organization responsible for the subsequent medical care of the patient.

*The asterisked items are key factors in the accreditation decision process.

MR.2.2.15.7 A final progress note may be substituted for the resume in the case of patients with problems of a minor nature who require less than a 48-hour period of hospitalization, and in the case of normal newborn infants and uncomplicated obstetric deliveries.

MR.2.2.15.7.1 The final progress note includes any instructions given to the patient and/or family.

MR.2.2.15.8 In the event of death, a summation statement is added to the record either as a final progress note or as a separate resume.

MR.2.2.15.8.1 The final note indicates the reason for admission, the findings and course in the hospital, and the events leading to death.

MR.2.2.15.9 When an autopsy is performed, provisional anatomic diagnoses are recorded in the medical record within three days, and the complete protocol is made part of the record within 60 days, unless exceptions for special studies are established by the medical staff.

Standard

MR.3   Medical records are confidential, secure, current, authenticated, legible, and complete.*

Required characteristics

MR.3.1   The medical record is the property of the

hospital and is maintained for the benefit of the patient, the medical staff, and the hospital.

MR.3.2 The hospital is responsible for safeguarding both the record and its informational content against loss, defacement, and tampering and from use by unauthorized individuals.

MR.3.2.1 Particular emphasis is given to protection from damage by fire or water.

MR.3.3 Written consent of the patient or his legally qualified representative is required for the release of medical information to persons not otherwise authorized to receive the information.

MR.3.3.1 This does not mean that written consent is required for the use of the medical record for

MR.3.3.1.1 automated data processing of designated information;

MR.3.3.1.2 use in activities concerned with the monitoring and evaluation of the quality and appropriateness of patient care;

MR.3.3.1.3 departmental review of work performance;

MR.3.3.1.4 official surveys for hospital compliance with accredition, regulatory, and licensing standards; or

MR.3.3.1.5 educational purposes and research programs.

MR.3.3.2 There is a written hospital and

medical staff policy that medical records may be removed from the hospital's jurisdiction and safekeeping only in accordance with a court order, subpoena, or statute.

MR.3.3.2.1 Any other restrictions on record removal are in addition to this basic requirement.

MR.3.4 When certain portions of the medical record are so confidential that extraordinary means are necessary to preserve their privacy, such as in the treatment of some psychiatric disorders, these portions may be stored separately, provided the complete record is readily available when required for current medical care or follow-up, review functions, or use in quality assurance activities.

MR.3.4.1 The medical record indicates that a portion has been filed elsewhere, in order to alert authorized reviewing personnel of its existence.

MR.3.5 The quality of the medical record depends in part on the timeliness, meaningfulness, authentication, and legibility of the informational content.*

MR.3.5.1 Entries in medical records are made only by individuals given this right as specified in hospital and medical staff policies.*

MR.3.5.2 All entries in the record are dated and authenticated, and a method is established to identify the authors of entries.*

MR.3.5.2.1 Identification may include written signatures, initials, or computer key.

MR.3.5.2.2 When rubber-stamp signatures are authorized, the individual whose signature the stamp represents places in the administrative offices of the hospital a signed statement to the effect that he is the only one who has the stamp and is the only one who will use it.

MR.3.5.2.2.1 There is no delegation of the use of such a stamp to another individual.

MR.3.5.3 The parts of the medical record that are the responsibility of the medical practitioner are authenticated by him.*

MR.3.5.3.1 For example, when non-physicians have been approved for such duties as taking medical histories and documenting some aspects of a physical examination, such information is appropriately authenticated by the physician responsible for the patient.

MR.3.5.4 When members of the house staff are involved in patient care, sufficient evidence is documented in the medical record to substantiate the active participation in, and supervision of, the patient's care by the attending physician responsible for the patient.*

---

*The asterisked items are key factors in the accreditation decision process.

MR.3.5.5 Any entries in the medical record by house staff or nonphysicians that require countersigning by supervisory or attending medical staff members are defined in the medical staff rules and regulations.*

MR.3.6 To avoid misinterpretation, symbols and abbreviations are used in the medical record only when they have been approved by the medical staff and when there is an explanatory legend available to those authorized to make entries in the medical record and to those who must interpret them.

MR.3.6.1 Each abbreviation or symbol has only one meaning.

MR.3.7 In the interest of accuracy, legibility, and responsibility, and when budgetary and personnel availability permit, medical record entries, when appropriate, are typed.

MR.3.7.1 Special consideration is given to the typing of radiology and pathology reports, operative reports, and clinical resumes.

MR.3.7.1.1 When transcription and filing of these medical records cannot be accomplished in a timely manner, written entries pertinent to the continuity of the patient care are recorded.

MR.3.8 Each clinical event, including the history and physical examination, is documented as soon as possible after its occurrence.*

*The asterisked items are key factors in the accreditation decision process.

CHAPTER 5

American Nurses' Association Standard I

◆

The collection of data about the health status of the client/patient is systematic and continuous. The data are accessible, communicated, and recorded.

RATIONALE

Comprehensive care requires complete and ongoing collection of data about the client/patient to determine the nursing care needs of the client/patient. All health status data about the client/patient must be available for all members of the health care team.

ASSESSMENT FACTORS

1. Health status data include:
    - Growth and development
    - Biophysical status
    - Emotional status
    - Cultural, religious, socioeconomic background
    - Performance of activities of daily living
    - Patterns of coping
    - Interaction patterns
    - Client's/patient's perception of and satisfaction with his health status
    - Client/patient health goals
    - Environment (physical, social, emotional, ecological)

- Available and accessible human and material resources
2. Data are collected from:
   - Client/patient, family, significant others
   - Health care personnel
   - Individuals within the immediate environment and/or the community
3. Data are obtained by:
   - Interview
   - Examination
   - Observation
   - Reading records, reports, etc.
4. There is a format for the collection of data which:
   - Provides for a systematic collection of data
   - Facilitates the completeness of data collection
5. Continuous collection of data is evident by:
   - Frequent updating
   - Recording of changes in health status
6. The data are:
   - Accessible on the client/patient records
   - Retrievable from record-keeping systems
   - Confidential when appropriate

From *Standards of Nursing Practice*, © 1973 by American Nurses' Association, Kansas City, MO. Reprinted with permission.

PART TWO

MEDICAL-SURGICAL CARE DOCUMENTATION GUIDE

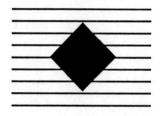

Acquired Immune Deficiency Syndrome (AIDS)

◆

1. **Assessment of the patient problem**

   Obtain subjective data from the patient, family, or
   caregiver(s)

2. **Associated nursing diagnoses**

   Activity intolerance
   Activity intolerance, high risk for
   Adjustment, impaired
   Airway clearance, ineffective
   Anxiety
   Body image disturbance
   Body temperature, altered, high risk for
   Bowel incontinence
   Cardiac output, decreased
   Coping, ineffective family: compromised
   Coping, ineffective family: disabling
   Coping, ineffective individual
   Disuse syndrome, high risk for
   Family processes, altered
   Fatigue
   Fear
   Fluid volume deficit
   Fluid volume deficit, high risk for
   Gas exchange, impaired
   Grieving, anticipatory
   Home maintenance management, impaired
   Infection, high risk for
   Knowledge deficit (e.g., diagnosis and treatment)
   Nutrition, altered: less than body requirements
   Oral mucous membrane, altered
   Pain
   Pain, chronic
   Powerlessness
   Protection, altered

Role performance, altered
Self-care deficit, bathing/hygiene
Self-care deficit, dressing/grooming
Self-care deficit, feeding
Self-care deficit, toileting
Sensory/perceptual alterations (specify) (visual,
auditory, kinesthetic, gustatory, tactile, olfactory)
Sexuality patterns, altered
Skin integrity, impaired
Skin integrity, impaired, high risk for
Social isolation
Spiritual distress (distress of the human spirit)
Swallowing, impaired
Thermoregulation, ineffective
Thought processes, altered
Tissue integrity, impaired
Tissue perfusion, altered (specify type) (renal, cerebral,
cardiopulmonary, gastrointestinal, peripheral)
Urinary elimination, altered patterns

3. **Examples of objective data for documentation**
    Height, weight
    General appearance
    Caloric intake
    Vital signs
    Level of consciousness
    Tears, crying
    IV solution, rate infusing, site description
    Hemoglobin, hematocrit
    Presence of catheter
    Functional mobility
    Diaphoresis
    Dyspnea
    History of illness (include dates)
    Lung sounds
    Intake and output
    Sputum production, frequency, amount, character
    Oxygen use

Bed position (e.g., semi-Fowler's)
Restlessness
Visitors present (specify)
Skin integrity
Lab results
Loose or liquid stools

4. **Examples of the assessment of the data**
   Unstable vital signs (e.g., BP high or low, febrile, change in vital signs)
   Alert, oriented x3
   Upset, depressed
   IV infusing
   Catheter patent, draining
   Pain
   Weight loss or gain
   Changes in lung sounds
   Infiltrated IV site evidenced by_____
   Patent catheter

5. **Examples of potential medical problems for this patient**
   Urinary tract infection
   Kaposi's sarcoma
   Pneumocystis carinii pneumonia
   Endocarditis
   Encephalitis
   Meningitis
   Myocarditis
   Tuberculosis
   Lymphomas
   Chorioretinitis
   Leukemias
   Squamous cell carcinomas of rectum and mouth
   Miscellaneous other protozoal, fungal, viral, or bacterial infections
   Allergic reactions to the antibiotic treatments

6. **Examples of the documentation of potential nursing interventions/actions**

Taught family, patient, or caregiver(s) care of patient

Daily weights and evaluation of weights

Pain, other symptoms assessed

Taught care of the bedridden patient

BP, respirations, pulse, temperature (specify route) being monitored q _____

Cardiovascular status assessed

Assessed hydration/nutritional status; evaluated for signs, symptoms of dehydration

Taught patient medication regimen

Teaching begun regarding diet as indicated; encouraging foods of choice

Pain control regimen of _____ implemented

Assessment of pulmonary, respiratory systems performed; specify for dyspnea, cough, sputum production, frequency, and amount

Taught patient oxygen therapy safety and use of oxygen therapy

Emotional support provided to patient, family/caregiver(s), and significant others

Oxygen on at _____ liters continuously or prn

Medications being monitored

Fluids high in electrolytes encouraged po

Emotional status assessed

Observed for signs of oral thrush (oral candidiasis)

Taught patient regarding elevation of edematous extremities and elevation of head of bed for comfort

Taught patient application and use of elastic support hose

Maintenance of hygiene and proper disposal of waste per facility policy; taught patient regarding same

Lab specimens for blood/urine/site culture(s) obtained per physician order(s)

Evaluated for lung changes

Changed or started IV solution of _____ at _____ (rate)

Comfort measures provided, including backrubs, hand massages

Changed catheter # _____, _____ cc per physician order(s)

Documented specific teaching accomplished and behavioral outcomes of that teaching

Medication being administered IM q _____ for _____ relief

Venipuncture as ordered for _____

Patient being given maximum assistance for all activities

Taught family regarding "universal precautions" or facility policy

Oral hygiene care provided

Reverse isolation as ordered

Culture of wound site performed

7. **Examples of the evaluations of the interventions/actions**

Temperature rechecked at _____ PM; now _____

No vomiting; patient reports no nausea

Patient no longer restless; validates pain relief

IV patent

Negative culture

Successful plan as evidenced by _____

Patient expresses comfort after repositioning; able to rest

Frequent (q _____) visits to patient for comfort, reassurance, reassessment

Patient able to verbalize wound regimen taught

8. **Other services that may be indicated and their associated interventions and goals/outcomes**

Nurse aide

Personal care

ADL assistance

Other duties

Goals:

Effective personal hygiene

ADL assistance provided

Patient clean and comfortable

Physical therapy

Evaluation
Strengthening exercises
Passive/active exercises
Transfer techniques
Pain management through positioning and assistive
devices
Bed mobility exercises
Management of sputum production/postural drainage
Goals:
> Increased function and mobility

Occupational therapy

Evaluation
Conservation-of-energy techniques
Adaptive or assistive devices as indicated
ADL training program
Teach alternative skills as indicated
Goals:
> Patient using conservation-of-energy techniques
> Quality of life improved through techniques being
> used

Chaplaincy

Spiritual support offered to patient,
family/caregiver(s)
Goals:
> Spiritual support provided to patient,
> family/caregiver(s)
> Referral to community spiritual resource(s) as
> indicated

Social work

Assessment of social and emotional factors
Counseling
Financial assistance
Housing or placement assistance as needed
Goals:
> Problems, resources identified

Discharge planning nurse/team
Home nursing care referral
Community resource referral(s)
Support referral(s)
Hospice referral
Goals:
  Community resource referral(s) as indicated

9. **Nursing goals and outcomes**
   Daily implementation of care plan, created within
   _____ hours of admission and updated and/or
   reevaluated q _____ hours or as indicated by patient's
   condition
   Symptom and infection control, patient pain-free,
   other symptoms controlled
   Functional independence, dependent on progression
   of process; comfort and curative and/or palliative care

10. **Potential discharge plans for this patient**
    Discharge to home
    Nursing home placement
    Return to home with home nursing services and
    rehabilitation therapies as indicated
    Patient death in facility with dignity and comfort,
    support by friends, family/caregiver(s)

Amputation

1. **Assessment of the patient problem**
   Obtain subjective data from the patient, family, or
   caregiver(s)

2. **Associated nursing diagnoses**
   Activity intolerance, high risk for
   Anxiety
   Body image disturbance
   Body temperature, altered, high risk for
   Decisional conflict (specify)
   Denial, ineffective
   Fear
   Grieving, anticipatory
   Infection, high risk for
   Injury, high risk for
   Mobility, impaired physical
   Nutrition, altered: high risk for more than body
   requirements
   Nutrition, altered: less than body requirements
   Nutrition, altered: more than body requirements
   Pain
   Pain, chronic
   Personal identity disturbance
   Role performance, altered
   Self-care deficit
   Sensory/perceptual alterations (specify) (visual,
   auditory, kinesthetic, gustatory, tactile, olfactory)
   Sexuality patterns, altered
   Skin integrity, impaired
   Tissue integrity, impaired
   Tissue perfusion, altered (peripheral)

3. **Examples of objective data for documentation**
   Tourniquet at bedside
   Drainage or bleeding and descriptives

Vital signs
Edema
Restlessness
Dressing description
Bedridden
Presence of Penrose drain
Needs maximum assistance to ambulate, transfer
Wound/stump site description (drainage or exudate
amount, color, and the specific care)

4. **Examples of the assessment of the data**
Wound healing progressing
Febrile
Changes in wound/stump incision site
Patient complaint of pain or pain relief
Safety concerns
Increased bleeding
Mobility restricted

5. **Examples of potential medical problems for this
patient**
Nonhealing
Hemorrhage
Wound site infection
Thrombophlebitis
Urinary tract infection
Debridement and infection
If patient has diabetes mellitus, complications
Pneumonia or other lung process
Healing complications
Impaction
Osteomyelitis

6. **Examples of the documentation of potential
nursing interventions/actions**
Documentation of the actual care of the wound
Documentation of the wound, including size, drainage
amount, color, etc.

Counseled patient regarding "phantom" pain or sensations

Communicated treatment plan/change implemented in nursing plan of care

Insulin increased to _____ units as ordered

Dressing regimen, frequency of wound changes; teaching begun with family/caregiver(s) regarding wound care regimen

Support provided to patient regarding major body image change

Patient's wound assessed

Wound cultured as ordered

Safety concerns assessed in patient with recent amputation

Taught patient to wrap stump site

Administered medication for pain

7. **Examples of the evaluations of the interventions/actions**

IV patent, infusing at rate of _____

Patient no longer restless; verbally validates pain relief

Temperature rechecked at _____PM; now _____

8. **Other services that may be indicated and their associated interventions and goals/outcomes**

Nurse aide

Personal care

ADL assistance

Patient clean and comfortable

Other duties

Goals:

Effective personal care provided

ADL assistance provided

Physical therapy

Evaluation

Therapeutic exercise regimen

Progressive strengthening program

Preprosthetic training

Temporary prosthetic construction and training
Transfer techniques
Donning and doffing of prosthesis
Stump conditioning
Gait training
Teach use of assistive devices as indicated
Teach stump hygiene, wrapping techniques, self examination of stump
Goals:

> Self-care of stump, including hygiene
>
> Return to self-ambulation with prosthetic or other device
>
> Compliance with exercise regimen taught
>
> Control of stump skin breakdown and liaison with prosthetist for adjustments to prosthesis
>
> Using assistive devices
>
> Shaping of stump; control of edema
>
> Reevaluation of periodic visits for follow-up and recommended adjustments

Occupational therapy

Evaluation
Safety assessment
Adaptive equipment evaluation
Provision of adaptive equipment for return to independent ADLs
Goals:

> Return to independence in ADLs using adaptive equipment

Chaplaincy

Spiritual support offered to patient, family/caregiver(s)
Goals:

> Spiritual support provided to patient, family/caregiver(s)
>
> Referral to community spiritual resource(s) as indicated

Social work

Assessment of emotional/social factors in patient with body image changes
Financial resource information to patient, family/caregiver(s)
Goals:
> Financial situation concerns referred to appropriate community resources
> Return home to self-care status
> New body image integration

Discharge planning nurse/team

Comprehensive patient evaluation and follow-up during length of stay
Communication of evaluation with other team members, patient, family/caregiver(s) as appropriate
Referral(s) to community resources
Goals:
> Comprehensive evaluation
> Referral(s) to community health resources

9. Nursing goals and outcomes

Daily implementation of care plan, created within _____ hours of admission and updated and/or reevaluated q _____ hours or as indicated by patient's condition
Return to self-care or status prior to hospitalization, pain-free with functional mobility and ambulation
Wound healing
Blood sugar stable for patient with diabetes mellitus
Patient infection-free
Patient returned to self-care status

10. Potential discharge plans for this patient

Return to home in community; self-care
Continued rehabilitation services for care of new prosthesis and stump site in home setting

Angina

◆

1. **Assessment of the patient problem**
   Obtain subjective data from the patient, family, or caregiver(s)

2. **Associated nursing diagnoses**
   Activity intolerance
   Activity intolerance, high risk for
   Anxiety
   Body image disturbance
   Breathing pattern, ineffective
   Cardiac output, decreased
   Constipation
   Coping, ineffective family: compromised
   Denial, ineffective
   Disuse syndrome, high risk for
   Diversional activity deficit
   Family processes, altered
   Fatigue
   Fear
   Fluid volume excess
   Gas exchange, impaired
   Grieving, anticipatory
   Home maintenance management, impaired
   Hopelessness
   Infection, high risk for
   Mobility, impaired physical
   Nutrition, altered: high risk for more than body
   requirements
   Nutrition, altered: less than body requirements
   Nutrition altered: more than body requirements
   Oral mucous membrane, altered
   Pain
   Pain, chronic
   Parenting, altered
   Parenting, altered, high risk for

Powerlessness
Role performance, altered
Self-care deficit, bathing/hygiene
Self-care deficit, dressing/grooming
Self-care deficit, feeding
Self-care deficit, toileting
Sexuality patterns, altered
Skin integrity, impaired
Skin integrity, impaired, high risk for
Sleep pattern disturbance
Social isolation
Spiritual distress (distress of the human spirit)
Tissue perfusion, altered (specify type) (renal, cerebral, cardiopulmonary, gastrointestinal, peripheral)
Urinary elimination, altered patterns

3. **Examples of objective data for documentation**
   Vital signs
   Level of consciousness
   Tears, crying
   Breath sounds
   IV solution, rate, site location and description
   Patient pointing to site of pain, duration of pain, description of pain
   Presence of urinary or other catheter(s)
   Weights
   Lung sounds
   Pedal edema, other measurements
   Amount, sites of fluid retention
   Skin color
   Last nitroglycerin dose (time, date)
   Use of antiembolus stockings
   Visitor's presence
   Family history (cardiac)
   Intake and output
   Oxygen use
   Fluid measurements
   Lab results

4. **Examples of the assessment of the data**
   Unstable vital signs
   Urinary catheter patent, draining
   Pain relief as indicated by _____
   High or low blood pressure
   Weight loss or gain
   Infiltrated IV site
   Dyspnea
   Fatigue
   Progress as demonstrated by _____
   Patient diuresing
   Change in vital signs
   Febrile
   Change in pulse from _____ to _____
   Alert, oriented x3
   Upset, depressed
   IV infusing
   Pain
   Change in breath sounds
   Patient progressing on cardiac rehabilitation program
   as evidenced by _____
   Family or caregiver(s) able to repeat cardiac discharge
   instructions

5. **Examples of potential medical problems for this patient**
   Pulmonary or other embolism
   Shock
   Thrombophlebitis
   Cerebrovascular accident
   Congestive heart failure
   Cardiac arrest
   Life-threatening arrhythmias
   Acute myocardial infarction
   Hypertension
   Electrolyte and fluid imbalances
   Pneumonia or other lung process

6. **Examples of the documentation of potential nursing interventions/actions**

Lung sounds assessed
Vital signs measured
Assessed patient for fluid retention
Taught patient conservation-of-energy techniques
Nitroglycerin administered and response noted
Assessment of amount, character, frequency, site(s) of pain performed; report to physician
Daily weights
Assessed for and monitored amount, sites of fluid retention
Measured intake and output
Taught patient relaxation techniques
Comfort measures provided, including backrubs, other massages
Obtained ECG strip and alerted physician to change
Measured specific gravity of urine
Checked for postural blood pressure changes
Maintained bed rest or other ordered activity level
Maintenance of bowel function; administered stool softeners as ordered
Administered medications as ordered (specify)
Patient teaching begun regarding medication regimen
Emotional support provided to patient and family
Antiembolus stockings applied
Ordered diet of _____ taught to patient and family

7. **Examples of the evaluations of the interventions/actions**

Patient comfortable, pain-free after nitroglycerin
ECG noted to be within normal limits for patient
Patient experiences no shortness of breath now
Arterial blood gases within normal range for patient
Temperature rechecked after antipyretic suppository administered; temperature now within normal range for patient
Caregiver now demonstrates correct procedure as taught by RN

8. **Other services that may be indicated and their associated interventions and goals/outcomes**

Nurse aide

Personal care
ADL assistance
Other duties
Goals:
> Personal care provided
> Patient clean and comfortable
> ADL assistance provided

Physical therapy

Evaluation
Begin cardiac rehabilitation program as ordered by physician
ROM
Progressive muscle strengthening program
Conditioning and endurance training
Goals:
> Increased mobility on discharge
> Family/caregiver(s) taught home program
> Safe use of assistive devices

Occupational therapy

Evaluation
Teach conservation-of-energy techniques
Modify ADL program as indicated
Goals:
> Patient using conservation-of-energy techniques taught
> Patient using adaptive equipment

Chaplaincy

Spiritual support offered to patient, family/caregiver(s)
Goals:
> Spiritual support provided to patient, family/caregiver(s)
> Referral to community spiritual resource(s) as indicated

Social work

Assessment of social and emotional factors impacting on health
Financial assistance
Referral(s) to community resources
Goals:
> Patient referred to community resources
> Discharge to appropriate setting

Discharge planning nurse/team

Comprehensive assessment
Referral(s) to identified resources
Home nursing care referral
Goals:
> Home nursing care referral accomplished
> Patient/family referred to needed resources
> Discharge to appropriate setting

9. **Nursing goals and outcomes**

    Daily implementation of care plan, created within
    _____ hours of admission and updated and/or
    reevaluated q _____ hours or as indicated by patient's
    condition
    Return to self-care or status prior to hospitalization,
    pain-free with functional mobility and ambulation
    Stable cardiac status, pain controlled, patient without
    anxiety
    Patient, family/caregiver(s) able to care for patient on
    discharge to home

10. **Potential discharge plans for this patient**

    Discharge to another facility
    Discharge to home with nursing and rehabilitative
    follow-up
    Other

Asthma

1. **Assessment of the patient problem**
   Obtain subjective data from the patient, family, or
   caregiver(s)

2. **Associated nursing diagnoses**
   Activity intolerance
   Activity intolerance, high risk for
   Anxiety
   Breathing pattern, ineffective
   Communication, impaired verbal
   Coping, family: potential for growth
   Fatigue
   Fear
   Fluid volume deficit, high risk for
   Gas exchange, impaired
   Health maintenance, altered
   Home maintenance management, impaired
   Injury, high risk for
   Knowledge deficit (diagnosis or treatment)
   Self-care deficit, bathing/hygiene
   Self-care deficit, dressing/grooming
   Self-care deficit, feeding
   Self-care deficit, toileting
   Sleep pattern disturbance

3. **Examples of objective data for documentation**
   Presence or absence of wheezing (NOTE: The absence
   can indicate worsening of condition)
   Vital signs
   Use of accessory muscles to breathe
   Cough
   Use of oxygen
   Presence of family/caregiver(s)
   Medications taken at home
   Results of arterial blood gases (ABGs), pulmonary

function tests, or x-ray
Difficulty talking due to severe shortness of breath

4. **Examples of the assessment of the data**
Tachycardia
Tachypnea
Unstable vital signs
Unable to sleep
IV infusing
Productive cough
Positive sputum culture

5. **Examples of potential medical problems for this patient**
Respiratory distress
Death
Acute bronchospasm
Cor pulmonale
Pneumonia
Pneumothorax

6. **Examples of the documentation of potential nursing interventions/actions**
Comprehensive baseline patient assessment performed
Administered nebulizer therapy as ordered
Patient maintained in upright position
Intake and output being monitored q _____ hours
Vital signs and patient's color, cough, and breath sounds being evaluated q _____
Physician notified of change in patient's status
Emotional support provided to patient and family
Patient's IV of _____ infusing at rate of _____ as ordered
Teaching begun with patient/caregiver regarding care of asthma
Oxygen on at _____ liters per nasal prongs/cannula
Patient offered fluids of choice as ordered to maintain 3000 cc/day intake

RN taught patient relaxation techniques
Patient teaching completed today; included
medications and their administration/application,
importance of rest, nutrition, exercise, fluids; factors
that precipitate an attack for patient and avoidance of
known factors, where possible; when to contact health
provider

7. **Examples of the evaluations of the
   interventions/actions**

   ABG results now _____, within normal range for
   patient
   Patient able to rest between planned interventions
   Patient no longer using accessory muscles and able to
   sleep
   Patient correctly demonstrated skill of _____ as
   taught by RN
   Patient free of signs, symptoms of infection

8. **Other services that may be indicated and their
   associated interventions and goals/outcomes**

   Nurse aide

   Personal care
   ADL assistance
   Other duties
   Goals:
       Effective personal care provided
       Patient clean and comfortable

   Physical therapy

   Evaluation
   Chest physical therapy
   Strengthening exercise regimen as tolerated
   Goals:
       Pulmonary goals achieved
       Discharged to home with prior mobility status

Patient, family demonstrate home exercise
program taught

Occupational therapy

Evaluation
Teach conservation-of-energy techniques
Goals:

Patient using conservation-of-energy techniques
taught
Patient can pace activities to subjectively have
more energy

Chaplaincy

Spiritual support offered to patient,
family/caregiver(s)
Goals:

Spiritual support provided to patient,
family/caregiver(s)

Social work

Assessment of emotional/social factors impacting on
health
Financial resource information to patient,
family/caregiver(s)
Referral(s) to identified community resources
Goals:

Problem identification and referral(s) to
appropriate community resources

Discharge planning nurse/team

Comprehensive patient evaluation
Communication of evaluation with other team
members
Goals:

Referral(s) to identified community resources

9. **Nursing goals and outcomes**

Daily implementation of care plan, created within
_____ hours of admission and updated and/or

reevaluated q _____ hours or as indicated by patient's condition
Return to self-care or status prior to hospitalization, pain-free with functional mobility and ambulation
Improved, adequate oxygen exchange
Daily adherence to treatment regimens taught
Stable status for respiratory and other systems
Adequate hydration/nutritional status
Patient, family/caregiver(s) able to demonstrate/verbalize care of patient with asthma

10. **Potential discharge plans for this patient**

   Nursing home placement for continued care of health problems
   Discharge to home with family able to care for patient
   Discharge to home with support of home nursing services

Bedbound Patient

1. **Assessment of the patient problem**
   Obtain subjective data from the patient, family, or caregiver(s)

2. **Associated nursing diagnoses**
   Aspiration, high risk for
   Body temperature, altered, high risk for
   Body image disturbance
   Bowel incontinence
   Constipation
   Disuse syndrome, high risk for
   Fatigue
   Fear
   Fluid volume deficit
   Gas exchange, impaired
   Incontinence, functional
   Infection, high risk for
   Injury, high risk for
   Mobility, impaired physical
   Nutrition, altered: less than body requirements
   Nutrition, altered: more than body requirements
   Oral mucous membrane, altered
   Pain
   Pain, chronic
   Parenting, altered
   Self-care deficit, bathing/hygiene
   Self-care deficit, dressing/grooming
   Self-care deficit, feeding
   Self-care deficit, toileting
   Sensory/perceptual alterations (specify) (visual,
   auditory, kinesthetic, gustatory, tactile, olfactory)
   Sexuality patterns, altered
   Skin integrity, impaired, high risk for
   Sleep pattern disturbance
   Social interaction, impaired

Social isolation
Spiritual distress (distress of the human spirit)
Swallowing, impaired
Unilateral neglect
Urinary elimination, altered patterns

3. **Examples of objective data for documentation**
   Vital signs
   Level of consciousness
   Loose or liquid stools
   Abdominal distention
   Cheyne-Stokes or irregular breathing pattern
   Hemiparesis
   Residual urine
   Slurred speech
   Temporal wasting
   Impaction present
   IV solution infusing at rate of _____
   Presence of urinary catheter
   Diaphoresis
   Restlessness
   Traction, casts
   Position
   Dyspnea
   Intake and output
   Weight
   Use of oxygen
   Skin color
   Presence of family/caregiver(s)
   Lab results
   Breath sounds

4. **Examples of the assessment of the data**
   Unstable vital signs (e.g., BP high or low, febrile, change in vital signs)
   Alert, oriented x3
   Unresponsive
   Impaction; patient unable to evacuate stool
   Upset, depressed, uncomfortable

Hemiparesis, quadriparesis
Patent urinary catheter
Traction in place at _____ lb
No swelling at cast site

5. **Examples of potential medical problems for this patient**
   Urinary tract infection
   Pneumonia or other lung process
   Thrombophlebitis
   Pulmonary embolism
   Cardiac complications
   Orthostatic hypotension
   Trauma (falls)

6. **Examples of the documentation of potential nursing interventions/actions**
   Patient monitored for signs, symptoms of infection
   Venipunctures obtained as ordered
   IV sites assessed for redness, signs of infiltration
   Reverse isolation maintained
   Fluid/hydration level monitored
   Repositioned patient
   Wound site(s) cultured
   Comfort measures provided, including backrubs, hand massages, soothing music of patient's choice
   Antiembolus hose applied
   Administered medication of _____ IM as ordered
   Obtained urine specimen for UA/C & S
   Assessed hydration/nutritional status
   Communication with family regarding patient's status and how they can assist, when appropriate
   Implemented skin care regimen to prevent decubitus
   Monitor bowel function
   Checked for impaction per physician order(s)
   Changed urinary catheter #_____, _____ cc per physician order(s)
   Oral hygiene care provided
   Joints placed in functional position

Emotional support provided to patient/family
Patient placed on air-fluidized therapy bed per
physician order(s)
Referral to enterostomal nurse therapist for skin care
consult

7. **Examples of the evaluations of the
   interventions/actions**

   Negative cultures
   Blood tests (e.g., WBC) within normal range for patient
   Afebrile
   No evidence of impaction
   Abdomen no longer distended
   Vital signs within normal range for patient
   Skin remains clear, dry, pink
   Urinary output within normal limits for patient
   Lung sounds clear
   Temperature rechecked at _____ PM; now _____
   Catheter patent; amber urine draining into bag
   Pain controlled now as evidenced by _____
   Caregiver demonstrated correct procedure of
   _____ as taught by RN

8. **Other services that may be indicated and their
   associated interventions and goals/outcomes**

   Nurse aide

   Personal care
   ADL assistance
   Other duties
   Goals:
   > Effective personal care provided
   > ADL assistance provided
   > Patient clean and comfortable

   Physical therapy

   Evaluation
   Therapeutic exercise regimen
   Chest physical therapy
   Bed mobility exercises as tolerated

ROM
Strengthening exercises
Passive and active exercises
Teach use of assistive devices as indicated
Goals:
>   Increased mobility
>   Maintenance of function
>   Prevention of complications in patient
>   Family/caregiver(s) able to demonstrate exercise
>   regimen

Occupational therapy

Evaluation
Splinting/positioning aids
Neuromuscular reeducation
Cognitive training
ADL techniques
Adaptive equipment evaluation
Teach conservation-of-energy techniques
Goals:
>   Splinting aids maintaining function
>   Increased coordination, strength

Speech-language pathology

Evaluation
Swallowing assessment
Speech dysphagia program
Alaryngeal speech
Goals:
>   Swallowing evaluation and subsequent tests
>   identified pathology; nutritional program
>   implemented; swallowing improved

Chaplaincy

Spiritual support offered to patient,
family/caregiver(s)
Goals:
>   Spiritual support provided to patient,
>   family/caregiver(s)

Social work

Assessment of emotional/social factors
Financial resource information to family/caregiver(s)
Personal emergency response system referral
Goals:
> Problem identification and referral(s) to
> appropriate resources
> Community resource referral(s)
> Personal emergency response system
> representative contacted

Discharge planning nurse/team

Comprehensive patient evaluation
Communication of evaluation with other team
members, patient, family/caregiver(s)
Referral(s) to community resources
Goals:
> Referral information communicated to nurse in
> facility to which patient is transferring
> Meeting with family/caregiver(s), other team
> members to facilitate continuity of care

9. Nursing goals and outcomes

Daily implementation of care plan, created within
_____ hours of admission and updated and/or
reevaluated q _____ hours or as indicated by patient's
condition
Return to self-care or status prior to hospitalization,
pain-free with functional mobility and ambulation
Skin is clear and intact
Heart rate, blood pressure, respirations are within an
acceptable range for this patient
Without infection
Stable weight achieved
Patient is afebrile
Lungs are clear

10. Potential discharge plans for this patient

Nursing home placement
Discharge to home with caregiver(s) trained and with
support of community home care services
Symptom-controlled death with dignity in inpatient
setting

Brain Tumor

◆

1. **Assessment of the patient problem**
   Obtain subjective data from the patient, family, or caregiver(s)

2. **Associated nursing diagnoses**
   Activity intolerance
   Activity intolerance, high risk for
   Airway clearance, ineffective
   Anxiety
   Aspiration, high risk for
   Body image disturbance
   Body temperature, altered, high risk for
   Bowel incontinence
   Breathing pattern, ineffective
   Communication, impaired verbal
   Constipation
   Disuse syndrome, high risk for
   Fatigue
   Fear
   Fluid volume deficit
   Fluid volume deficit, high risk for
   Fluid volume excess
   Gas exchange, impaired
   Grieving, anticipatory
   Grieving, dysfunctional
   Growth and development, altered
   Home maintenance management, impaired
   Hyperthermia
   Hypothermia
   Incontinence, total
   Infection, high risk for
   Injury, high risk for
   Mobility, impaired physical
   Nutrition, altered: less than body requirements
   Oral mucous membrane, altered

Pain
Pain, chronic
Role performance, altered
Self-care deficit, bathing/hygiene
Self-care deficit, dressing/grooming
Self-care deficit, feeding
Self-care deficit, toileting
Sensory/perceptual alterations (specify) (visual, auditory, kinesthetic, gustatory, tactile, olfactory)
Sexual dysfunction
Skin integrity, impaired
Skin integrity, impaired, high risk for
Sleep pattern disturbance
Spiritual distress (distress of the human spirit)
Swallowing, impaired
Thought processes, altered
Trauma, high risk for
Urinary elimination, altered patterns

3. **Examples of objective data for documentation**
   Vital signs
   The time the patient returned from radiation or other therapy
   Level of consciousness
   Slurred speech
   Hemiparesis
   IV solution of _____
   Presence of urinary or other catheter(s)
   Loose or liquid stools
   Restlessness
   Position
   Presence of family/caregiver(s)
   Seizure activity
   Pupil response
   Vomiting

4. **Examples of the assessment of the data**
   Cerebral swelling
   Unstable vital signs

Patient deterioration
Alert, oriented x3
Patient exhibiting signs of increased intracranial
pressure

5. **Examples of potential medical problems for this patient**
   Varied: tumor/site/type dependent
   Metastases
   Deafness
   Blindness
   Deep vein thrombosis
   Pulmonary emboli
   CVA
   Neurological deficits
   Seizures
   Pneumonia
   Meningitis
   Wound site or other infection(s)

6. **Examples of the documentation of potential nursing interventions/actions**
   Supportive care provided
   Checked incision site for bleeding
   Monitored for cerebrospinal fluid leakage
   Assessed site for signs of infection
   Fluid intake being monitored closely (fluids may be restricted)
   Evaluated for neurological changes or deficits
   Intake and output being monitored
   Assessed for signs of overhydration
   Assessed for symptoms of increased intracranial pressure (ICP)
   Comfort measures provided
   Monitored for fluid retention
   Daily weights
   Safety measures implemented for patient with seizures
   Administered steroids per facility protocol
   Evaluated breath sounds through auscultation

Pain assessment and documentation performed
Offering a high-protein diet and foods of patient's
choice as tolerated

7. **Examples of the evaluations of the interventions/actions**

Stable weight
Blood tests within normal range for patient
Afebrile
Catheter patent
Patient no longer restless
Seizure activity decreased

8. **Other services that may be indicated and their associated interventions and goals/outcomes**

Nurse aide

Personal care
ADL assistance
Other duties
Goals:
    Effective personal care provided
    Comfort measures provided
    ADL assistance provided
    Patient clean and comfortable

Physical therapy

Evaluation
Strengthening exercises
Bed mobility exercises as tolerated
Teach patient, family/caregiver(s) exercises as
tolerated
Teach use of assistive devices as indicated
Proprioception-neuromuscular facilitation (PNF)
Teach orthotic care
Assess gait safety
Therapeutic exercise regimen
Teach regarding transfer training
Gait training

Gait training with walker or other assistive devices
Goals:
> Function maintained
> Safe use of assistive device
> Family/caregiver(s) able to assist in safe transfer
> Prevention of further complications in at-risk patient
> Family/caregiver(s) able to demonstrate exercise regimen taught
> Increased mobility

Occupational therapy

Evaluation
Adaptive equipment evaluation
Conservation-of-energy techniques
Cognitive training
Goals:
> Patient able to use conservation-of-energy techniques taught
> Effective use of ADL training skills

Speech-language pathology

Evaluation
Swallowing assessment
Speech dysphagia program
Goals:
> Patient able to communicate
> Family taught and demonstrates techniques to safely facilitate swallowing

Chaplaincy

Spiritual support offered to patient, family/caregiver(s)
Goals:
> Spiritual support provided to patient, family/caregiver(s)
> Referral to community spiritual resource(s) as indicated

Social work

Assessment of emotional/social factors
Financial resource information to patient,
family/caregiver(s)
Goals:
    Psychosocial support
    Problem and resource identification

Discharge planning nurse/team

Comprehensive patient evaluation
Communication of evaluation(s) to patient, family/
caregiver(s), other team members
Referral(s) to community health resources as
appropriate
Goals:
    Referral(s) to appropriate community health
    resources
    Hospice or home care referral based on prognosis
    and patient preference

9. Nursing goals and outcomes

Daily implementation of care plan, created within
    _____ hours of admission and updated and/or
reevaluated q _____ hours or as indicated by patient's
condition
Return to self-care or status prior to hospitalization,
pain-free with functional mobility and ambulation
Patient without thrombophlebitis
Pain and other symptoms controlled
Comfort maintained through death with dignity
Patient without seizures, or seizures controlled
Patient, family/caregiver(s) able to participate in care
programs
Nutritional and fluid status stabilized for patient
Patient infection-free and afebrile
Skin is clear and intact
Supportive care provided to patient and family

10. **Potential discharge plans for this patient**

    Discharge to home with appropriate community
    health resources

    Death in inpatient facility with dignity and with
    patient, family/caregiver(s) as involved as possible

Cancer Care

1. **Assessment of the patient problem**

   Obtain subjective data from the patient, family, or caregiver(s)

2. **Associated nursing diagnoses**

   Activity intolerance
   Activity intolerance, high risk for
   Adjustment, impaired
   Airway clearance, ineffective
   Anxiety
   Aspiration, high risk for
   Body image disturbance
   Body temperature, altered, high risk for
   Breathing pattern, ineffective
   Cardiac output, decreased
   Constipation
   Coping, ineffective family: compromised
   Denial, ineffective
   Disuse syndrome, high risk for
   Family processes, altered
   Fatigue
   Fear
   Grieving, anticipatory
   Home maintenance management, impaired
   Infection, high risk for
   Injury, high risk for
   Knowledge deficit (e.g., diagnosis and treatment/options)
   Mobility, impaired physical
   Nutrition, altered: less than body requirements
   Pain
   Pain, chronic
   Parenting, altered
   Powerlessness
   Role performance, altered

Self-care deficit, bathing/hygiene
Self-care deficit, dressing/grooming
Self-care deficit, feeding
Self-care deficit, toileting
Sensory/perceptual alterations (specify) (visual, auditory, kinesthetic, gustatory, tactile, olfactory)
Sexuality patterns, altered
Skin integrity, impaired
Skin integrity, impaired, high risk for
Social interaction, impaired
Social isolation
Spiritual distress (distress of the human spirit)
Swallowing, impaired
Thought processes, altered
Tissue integrity, impaired
Urinary elimination, altered patterns
Urinary retention

3. **Examples of objective data for documentation**
   Blood or urine culture results
   Impaction noted on exam
   Patient febrile at _____
   Vital signs
   Level of consciousness
   Tears
   IV solution, rate ordered, site description
   Presence of urinary or other catheter(s)
   Urine: color, amount, odor
   Restlessness
   Lung sounds
   Dyspnea
   Patient's position (semi-Fowler's, etc.)
   Intake and output
   Presence of visitors
   Daily weights
   Lab results
   Loose stools
   Use of oxygen
   Use of assistive devices (walker, cane)

Positive urine, blood culture for _____ ; patient
began on _____
Impaction removed manually
Spoke with physician at _____ AM/PM regarding

_____

Pulse irregular at _____

4. **Examples of the assessment of the data**
Unstable vital signs (e.g., BP high or low, febrile,
changes in vital signs)
Alert, oriented x3
Upset/depressed
Crying
IV infusing
Patent catheter
Changes in lung sounds
Pain relief—patient resting
Weight loss or gain
Impaction

5. **Examples of potential medical problems for this patient**
Urinary tract infection
Pneumonia or other lung process
Thrombophlebitis
Impaction
Metastases
Malignant ascites
Radiation enteritis
Radiation myelitis
Leukopenia
Trauma (falls)

6. **Examples of the documentation of potential nursing interventions/actions**
Taught family or caregiver(s) care of patient
Assessed bowel regimen and implemented program as
needed

Assessed pain, other symptoms

Taught care of the bedridden patient

Assessed cardiovascular, pulmonary, and respiratory status

Assessed hydration/nutritional status

Taught new pain or symptom control medication regimen

Diet counseling initiated for patient with anorexia

Checked for and removed impaction

Taught care of condom catheter or indwelling catheter as indicated

Taught feeding tube care to family

Taught caregiver(s) symptom control and relief measures of _____

Assessed patient's and family's coping skills

Assessed weight as ordered

Measured abdominal girth for ascites and edema, documented sites, and recorded amount

Oxygen on at _____ liters per _____

Assessed mental status and sleep disturbance changes

Obtained venipuncture prn as ordered

Taught new medications and effects

Administered ordered medications for pain control

Taught catheter care to caregiver(s)

Taught family/caregiver(s) injection techniques and assessed for complications

Assessed amount and frequency of urinary output

Taught family regarding safety, specifically

_____

Taught patient and family about conservation-of-energy techniques

Emotional support provided to patient and family

Monitored for signs, symptoms of infection(s)

Reverse isolation being maintained as ordered

Hand, back massages, other comfort measures provided to patient

Supportive care provided to patient

7. **Examples of the evaluations of the interventions/actions**

Negative (or positive) cultures
Blood tests (e.g., WBC) within normal range for patient
Afebrile
No evidence of impaction now
Abdomen no longer distended
Catheter patent
IV infusing at rate of _____
Patient verbally validates pain relief
Successful plan as evidenced by _____
Patient expresses comfort after repositioning; able to rest
Patient participating in care by _____

8. **Other services that may be indicated and their associated interventions and goals/outcomes**

Nurse aide

Personal care
ADL assistance
Other duties
Goals:
> Effective personal care provided
> ADL assistance provided
> Patient clean and comfortable

Physical therapy

Evaluation
Therapeutic exercise program
Bed mobility exercises
Chest physical therapy
ROM
Teach orthotic care and ADL to patient, family/caregiver(s)
Teach use of assistive devices
Teach safe transfer techniques to patient, family/caregiver(s)
Goals:
> Increased mobility as evidenced by _____
> Function maintained; patient able to use assistive devices

Patient/caregiver(s) taught exercise regimen

Occupational therapy

Evaluation
Adaptive assistance devices as indicated
ADL training
Conservation-of-energy techniques
Functional mobility
Upper extremity therapeutic exercise and activities
Cognitive perceptual deficit training
Goals:
> Patient using adaptive devices
> Patient taught conservation-of-energy techniques
> Other services as appropriate for patient to improve and/or maintain quality of life

Speech-language pathology

Comprehensive evaluation
Swallowing evaluation as indicated
Teach and develop a communication program
Goals:
> Patient able to swallow safely
> Patient able to communicate and be understood

Chaplaincy

Spiritual support offered to patient,
family/caregiver(s)
Goals:
> Spiritual support provided to patient,
> family/caregiver(s)
> Referral to community spiritual resource(s) as indicated

Social work

Assessment of emotional/social factors impacting on patient and family
Financial resource information as needed
Referral of patient/family to community support services (e.g., "I Can Cope," classes of the American Cancer Society, other cancer support groups)

Goals:
>   Community resources identified
>   Problem resolution of identified problems

Discharge planning nurse/team
Comprehensive patient evaluation
Communication of evaluation with other team
members, patient, family/caregiver(s)
Referral(s) to community resources
Goals:
>   Comprehensive evaluation identified posthospital
>   needs
>   Referral to home care program
>   Referral to hospice program

9. Nursing goals and outcomes
Daily implementation of care plan, created within
_____ hours of admission and updated and/or
reevaluated q _____ hours or as indicated by patient's
condition
Return to self-care or status prior to hospitalization,
pain-free with functional mobility and ambulation
Pain, other symptoms controlled
Comfort achieved
Patient or caregiver(s) able to care for patient
Patient without infection
Patient is afebrile
Side-effects of radiation, chemotherapy controlled

10. Potential discharge plans for this patient
Discharged when goals achieved
Death, with symptoms controlled, in facility setting
Referral to home; family/caregiver(s) able to care for
patient
Referral back to community; self-care
Discharge to home with support of hospice
Discharge to home with home nursing services follow-
up for identified nursing needs

Cataract Care

1. **Assessment of the patient problem**
   Obtain subjective data from the patient, family, or
   caregiver(s)

2. **Associated nursing diagnoses**
   Anxiety
   Fear
   Injury, high risk for
   Pain
   Self-care deficit, bathing/hygiene
   Self-care deficit, dressing/grooming
   Self-care deficit, feeding
   Self-care deficit, toileting
   Sensory/perceptual alterations (specify) (visual,
   auditory, kinesthetic, gustatory, tactile, olfactory)
   Trauma, high risk for

3. **Examples of objective data for documentation**
   Visible opacities
   Vital signs
   Use of contact lenses or glasses
   Visitor's presence
   Patient's position

4. **Examples of the assessment of the data**
   Unstable vital signs
   Patient avoiding lying on the side that has been
   operated on, as taught by RN
   Severe visual deficit

5. **Examples of potential medical problems for this
   patient**
   Acute glaucoma
   Hemorrhage

Dehiscence
Systemic effects of topical ophthalmic medications
Iris prolapse
Infection
Falls/trauma

6. **Examples of the documentation of potential nursing interventions/actions**

Orientation given on physical layout of patient's room
Explanation of procedure and usual postoperative course given
Patient taught about increased light sensitivity
Patient cautioned to avoid straining or lifting activities
Visual acuity assessed
Patient assigned to quiet room postoperatively
Vital signs monitored
Pain medication administered
Antiemetic given to patient after complaint of nausea
Dressings examined for amount of bloody exudate
Head of bed positioned at 30-degree angle
Eye patch applied
Patient cautioned to avoid rubbing eyes
Patient assisted with all ADL
Taught patient/family about avoidance of activities causing increased ocular pressure
Taught patient/family eye care techniques
Taught patient/family administration/installation procedures for drops/ointments
Monitored blood pressure readings

7. **Examples of the evaluations of the interventions/actions**

Patient pain-free after administration of ordered analgesic
Amount of bloody drainage on dressing reported to physician
Patient experiencing no nausea after administration of ordered antiemetic
Patient comfortable after backrub given

Family member can demonstrate what nurse has
taught

8. **Other services that may be indicated and their
associated interventions and goals/outcomes**

Nurse aide

Personal care
ADL assistance
Other duties
Goals:
Effective personal care provided; patient verbalizes
feeling of comfort
Assistance with all ADL

Chaplaincy

Spiritual support offered to patient,
family/caregiver(s)
Goals:
Spiritual support provided to patient,
family/caregiver(s)
Referral to community spiritual resource(s) as
indicated

Social work

Assessment of emotional/social factors impacting on
health
Financial assistance
Referral(s) to resources as identified by needs
assessment
Goals:
Evaluation
Problem identification and referral(s) as
appropriate

Discharge planning nurse/team

Comprehensive patient evaluation
Communication of plan with patient, family, other
team members
Referral(s) to identified community resources

9. **Nursing goals and outcomes**

   Daily implementation of care plan, created within
   _____ hours of admission and updated and/or
   reevaluated q _____ hours or as indicated by patient's
   condition
   Return to self-care or status prior to hospitalization,
   pain-free with functional mobility and ambulation
   Patient/family/caregiver(s) able to care for patient on
   discharge
   Infection-free
   Pain controlled

10. **Potential discharge plans for this patient**

    Discharge to home with family able to care for patient
    Discharge to nursing home for support, ADL
    retraining
    Discharge to home; self-care

Cerebrovascular Accident

◆

1. **Assessment of the patient problem**

   Obtain subjective data from the patient, family, or caregiver(s)

2. **Associated nursing diagnoses**

   Activity intolerance
   Airway clearance, ineffective
   Anxiety
   Aspiration, high risk for
   Body image disturbance
   Body temperature, altered, high risk for
   Bowel incontinence
   Breathing pattern, ineffective
   Cardiac output, decreased
   Communication, impaired verbal
   Constipation
   Coping, ineffective family: compromised
   Denial, ineffective
   Disuse syndrome, high risk for
   Diversional activity deficit
   Family processes, altered
   Fatigue
   Fear
   Fluid volume deficit, high risk for
   Fluid volume excess
   Gas exchange, impaired
   Home maintenance management, impaired
   Hopelessness
   Incontinence, total
   Infection, high risk for
   Injury, high risk for
   Mobility, impaired physical
   Nutrition, altered: high risk for more than body requirements
   Nutrition, altered: less than body requirements

Nutrition, altered: more than body requirements
Oral mucous membrane, altered
Pain
Pain, chronic
Powerlessness
Self-care deficit, bathing/hygiene
Self-care deficit, dressing/grooming
Self-care deficit, feeding
Self-care deficit, toileting
Sensory/perceptual alterations (specify) (visual, auditory, kinesthetic, gustatory, tactile, olfactory)
Sexuality patterns, altered
Skin integrity, impaired, high risk for
Spiritual distress (distress of the human spirit)
Swallowing, impaired
Thought processes, altered
Tissue perfusion, altered (specify type) (renal, cerebral, cardiopulmonary, gastrointestinal, peripheral)
Unilateral neglect
Urinary elimination, altered patterns
Urinary retention

3. **Examples of objective data for documentation**
   Vital signs
   Level of consciousness
   Slurred speech
   Tears, crying
   Hemiparesis, unable to move LLE or RLE, etc.
   Asymmetry in facial features
   IV solution, rate ordered, site description
   Urinary catheter, color, amount, odor, sediment
   Lung sounds

4. **Examples of the assessment of the data**
   Unstable vital signs (e.g., BP high or low, febrile, change in vital signs)
   Alert, oriented x 3
   Upset, depressed
   IV infusing

Patent urinary catheter
Change in lung sounds

5. **Examples of potential medical problems for this patient**
   Pulmonary embolism
   Urinary tract infection
   Pneumonia or other lung process
   Thrombophlebitis
   Impaction
   Aspiration
   Another CVA

6. **Examples of the documentation of the potential nursing interventions/actions**
   BP, respirations, pulse, temperature (specify route) being measured q _____
   Level of consciousness being evaluated q _____
   Emotional support provided to patient and family
   Proper positioning of affected extremity
   Bowel regimen implemented to prevent constipation/impaction
   Hydration/nutritional status being monitored
   Taught patient regarding medication regimen and possible side effects
   Changed (or started) IV solution of _____, _____ cc at _____
   Obtained urine specimen for UA/C & S; sent to lab per physician order(s)
   Assessed lung, cardiovascular status
   Changed catheter # _____, _____ cc per physician order(s)
   Antiembolus hose applied per physician order(s)
   Bowel regimen, recommended by family, implemented

7. **Examples of the evaluations of the interventions/actions**
   Temperature rechecked at _____ PM; now _____

Family sitting with patient; patient not crying
Affected _____ arm propped with pillows
Drinking _____ cc during 8-hour shift
Catheter patent; yellow urine draining into drainage
bag
IV patent; site without problem (describe site)

8. **Other services that may be indicated and their
   associated interventions and goals/outcomes**

   Nurse aide
   Personal care
   ADL assistance
   Other duties
   Goals:
       Patient clean and comfortable

   Physical therapy
   Evaluation
   Therapeutic exercise regimen
   Teach regarding transfer training
   Gait training
   Gait training with cane or other assistive devices
   Strengthening exercises
   Home program and maintenance therapy
   Chest physical therapy program
   Teach orthotic care, orthotic ADL
   Gait safety assessment
   Passive exercise regimen
   Active assistive exercise regimen
   Goals:
       Increased mobility
       Safe use of assistive devices
       Trained in maintenance program including ROM,
       strength, coordination, and safety

   Occupational therapy
   Evaluation
   ADL training program
   Muscle reeducation

Upper extremity therapeutic exercises and activities
Swallowing evaluation
Independent bathing or other ADL
Recommendation of food textures to decrease risk of
aspiration
Teach alternative bathing, dressing, feeding skills
Evaluate need for splints and orthoses
Assistive device evaluation
Cognitive-perceptual deficits retraining
Functional mobility
Therapeutic exercises to increase strength,
coordination and sensation
Goals:
> ADL retraining provided
> Patient able to swallow safely
> Using adaptive equipment

Speech-language pathology

Evaluation
Video swallowing test and evaluation
Alaryngeal speech
Food texture recommendations
Language processing
Speech dysphagia instruction program
Continue therapy to increase articulation, proficiency,
verbal expression
Lip, tongue, and facial exercises to improve
swallowing and vocal skills
Word fluency exercises
Short-term memory skills
Establish home maintenance program
Goals:
> Patient able to communicate and swallow safely

Chaplaincy

Spiritual support offered to patient,
family/caregiver(s)
Support offered to elderly spouse or caregiver
Goals:
> Spiritual support provided to patient,
> family/caregiver(s)

Social work

Assessment of social and emotional factors
Counseling
Financial assistance
Nursing home placement assistance
Arrange for meal program(s)
Goals:

> Problem identification
> Referral(s) to appropriate resources
> Community referral(s)
> Personal emergency response system referral initiated

Discharge planning nurse/team

Home nursing care referral for follow-up nursing needs and/or rehabilitative services
Personal emergency response system referral
Goals:

> Referral information communicated to nurse in facility to which patient is to be transferred
> Meeting with family/caregiver(s) and other team members to facilitate continuity of care planning
> Referral to community home nursing services for continued rehabilitative care

9. **Nursing goals and outcomes**

   Daily implementation of care plan, created within _____ hours of admission and updated and/or reevaluated q _____ hours or as indicated by patient's condition or facility protocol
   Able to perform ADLs and return home with a maximum of function

10. **Potential discharge plans for this patient**

    Discharge to home; goals achieved, patient functional
    Nursing home placement
    Return to home with continued nursing and rehabilitation therapy at home

Chronic Obstructive Pulmonary Disease

◆

1. Assessment of the patient problem

Obtain subjective data from the patient, family, or caregiver(s)

2. Associated nursing diagnoses

Activity intolerance
Activity intolerance, high risk for
Airway clearance, ineffective
Anxiety
Aspiration, high risk for
Body temperature, altered, high risk for
Breathing pattern, ineffective
Fatigue
Fear
Gas exchange, impaired
Infection, high risk for
Mobility, impaired physical
Nutrition, altered: less than body requirements
Oral mucous membrane, altered
Pain
Pain, chronic
Self-care deficit, bathing/hygiene
Self-care deficit, dressing/grooming
Self-care deficit, feeding
Self-care deficit, toileting
Sexuality patterns, altered
Sleep pattern disturbance
Swallowing, impaired

3. Examples of objective data for documentation

Patient smokes _____ packs of cigarettes a day (began
19__)
Specific use and parameters of oxygen use
Results of chest x-ray
Results of ABGs, other diagnostic information

Presence of rales, rhonchi
Presence and character of cough, sputum production
Positive PPD
Mouth breathing
Use of assistive devices
Presence of family/caregiver(s)

4. **Examples of the assessment of the data**
   Positive blood cultures
   Febrile
   Unstable vital signs
   Anxiety decreased after questions
   answered/explanations given
   Weight loss of _____ lb since last admission on
   _____
   Patient diuresing after begun on new medication
   Pain in chest when coughing or deep breathing
   Upset, uncomfortable
   Alert, anxious
   Physician notified of change
   Decreased output this hour of _____ cc
   Change in breath sounds

5. **Examples of potential medical problems for this patient**
   Pneumonia
   Pneumothorax
   Respiratory failure
   Cor pulmonale
   Infection(s)
   Electrolyte imbalances
   Other system processes

6. **Examples of the documentation of potential nursing interventions/actions**
   Physician called regarding change in patient condition

Baseline patient assessment performed
Administered ordered antibiotic of _____
Administered nebulizer therapy with bronchodilator
Vital signs being monitored q _____ hours
Comfort measure of back massage provided
Care being planned, when possible, with spans of rest
periods for patient comfort
Evaluated breath sounds: site(s) wheezing, rhonchi,
other clinical findings
Assessed hydration/nutritional status
Patient/family taught conservation-of-energy
techniques
Patient/family taught and able to participate in care
where possible
RN met with home care nurse who has been seeing
this patient in the home to facilitate continuity of care
Venipuncture obtained as ordered
Patient given antiemetic after complaint of nausea
Assessed for signs, symptoms of infection
Patient suctioned of copious secretions
Sputum sample obtained and sent to lab for culture
and sensitivity

7. **Examples of the evaluations of the
   interventions/actions**

   Pain relief after administration of ordered medication
   Patient able to rest now between planned interventions
   Patient demonstrated correct breathing exercise as
   taught by RN
   ABGs now within normal range for patient
   Family able to verbalize and demonstrate skills taught
   by RN
   Patient intake has improved with offering of smaller,
   more frequent meals
   Temperature within normal range for patient this AM
   Patient's weight remains stable at _____

Bowel regimen effective; patient had bowel movement
this AM
Decreased wheezing on auscultation

8. **Other services that may be indicated and their
associated interventions and goals/outcomes**

Nurse aide

Personal care
ADL assistance
Other duties
Goals:
    Effective personal care provided
    Patient clean and comfortable

Physical therapy

Evaluation
Chest physical therapy
Breathing exercises and instructions
Teach coughing techniques
Therapeutic exercise regimen, if tolerated
Bed mobility exercises
Strengthening exercises
Goals:
    Pulmonary program goals achieved
    Increased patient mobility
    Discharged to prior mobility status
    Patient, family/caregiver(s) able to demonstrate
    home exercise regimen taught

Occupational therapy

Evaluation
ADL training
Teach conservation-of-energy techniques
Upper extremity exercises and activities
Compensatory techniques
Teach diaphragmatic/pursed lip breathing techniques
Goals:
    Patient using new skills taught
    Return to ADL prior to hospital stay
    Functional mobility

Chaplaincy

Spiritual support offered to patient,
family/caregiver(s)
Goals:
> Spiritual support provided to patient,
> family/caregiver(s)
> Referral to community spiritual resource(s) as
> indicated

Social work

Assessment of social/emotional factors impacting on
health
Financial resource information as requested
Referral(s) to community support groups
Goals:
> Problem identification and referral(s) to
> community resources

Discharge planning nurse/team

Comprehensive patient evaluation
Communication of outcome(s) to other team members
Referral(s) to identified community resources
Goals:
> Nursing home placement with follow-up care and
> therapy services

9. **Nursing goals and outcomes**

   Daily implementation of care plan, created within
   _____ hours of admission and updated and/or
   reevaluated q _____ hours or as indicated by patient's
   condition or facility protocol
   Return to self-care or status prior to hospitalization,
   pain-free with functional mobility and ambulation
   Stable respiratory status for patient
   Improved oxygen exchange
   Afebrile
   Patient or family able to implement regimens taught in
   hospital
   Adequate hydration/nutritional status
   Medications regulated

10. Potential discharge plans for this patient

Discharge to home; self-care status with
patient/family able to care for patient
Discharge to home with support of home nursing
services for continued skilled care and therapy services
Symptom-controlled death in inpatient setting

Congestive Heart Failure

1. **Assessment of the patient problem**
   Obtain subjective data from the patient, family, or caregiver(s)

2. **Associated nursing diagnoses**
   Activity intolerance
   Anxiety
   Breathing pattern, ineffective
   Cardiac output, decreased
   Fatigue
   Fear
   Fluid volume excess
   Gas exchange, impaired
   Powerlessness
   Self-care deficit, bathing/hygiene
   Self-care deficit, dressing/grooming
   Self-care deficit, feeding
   Self-care deficit, toileting
   Skin integrity, impaired
   Sleep pattern disturbance
   Spiritual distress (distress of the human spirit)

3. **Examples of objective data for documentation**
   Dyspnea
   Vomiting
   Vital signs
   Oxygen use
   Family/caregiver(s) accompanying patient
   Abdominal distention
   Results of ABGs, chest x-rays, other diagnostic data
   Weight
   Diaphoresis
   Edema (general, peripheral)
   Increased jugular distention

4. **Examples of the assessment of the data**
   Unstable vital signs
   Alert, anxious, confused
   IV patent
   Physician notified of change
   Decreased urinary output of _____ this hour
   Patient eating foods of choice with diet regimen
   Skin integrity maintained; patient on air-fluidized bed

5. **Examples of potential medical problems for this patient**
   Pulmonary edema
   Skin breakdown
   Electrolyte imbalance
   Drug toxicity
   Ascites
   Pleural effusion
   Increased work of heart
   Decreased blood supply to vital organs

6. **Examples of the documentation of potential nursing interventions/actions**
   Comprehensive baseline assessment performed
   Patient placed in high-Fowler's position
   Position of patient being changed q 2 hours
   Evaluated and reported results of ABGs
   Hemodynamic indicators being monitored as ordered
   Skin integrity assessed; continue repositioning patient q 2 hours
   Patient placed on alternating-pressure mattress
   Antiembolus stockings applied
   Patient on low-sodium diet; good nutrition reinforced and taught to spouse
   Oxygen administered per orders
   Medication (_____) administered
   Patient being weighed daily
   Patient teaching: medication education continuing
   Comfort measures provided
   Emotional support provided to patient, family/caregiver(s)

Explanation of all procedures/therapies given to patient/family

7. **Examples of the evaluations of the interventions/actions**

   Pain relief expressed after administration of analgesic
   Lab value of _____, now within normal range for patient
   Patient able to rest between planned interventions
   Weight decreased from yesterday (specify date)
   Skin integrity remains intact; continue with q 2 hour regimen
   Patient able to rest after backrub
   Family demonstrating understanding of diet teaching: brought in low-salt favorite foods

8. **Other services that may be indicated and their associated interventions and goals/outcomes**

   Nurse aide

   Personal care
   ADL assistance
   Other duties
   Goals:
   > Effective personal care provided
   > Patient clean and comfortable
   > Assistance with ADL provided

   Chaplaincy

   Spiritual support offered to patient, family/caregiver(s)
   Goals:
   > Spiritual support provided to patient, family/caregiver(s)
   > Referral to community spiritual resource(s) as indicated

   Social work

   Assessment of social/emotional factors impacting on health

Counseling
Financial assistance
Referral(s) to resources as identified by needs assessment
Goals
> Resources identified and referral(s) made to community programs

Dietitian

Proper nutrition, low-sodium diet, potassium
Purchasing and preparation of meals
Goals:
> Patient being provided with proper diet

Discharge planning nurse/team

Comprehensive evaluation of patient's needs
Home nursing care referral
Goals:
> Discharge to home; returned to self-care status

9. **Nursing goals and outcomes**

Daily implementation of care plan, created within _____ hours of admission and updated and/or reevaluated q _____ hours or as indicated by patient's condition
Return to self-care or status prior to hospitalization, pain-free with functional mobility and ambulation
Decreased anxiety
Stable cardiovascular status—effective perfusion occurring
Decreased fluid overload
Medications regulated
Patient able to care for self, or family/caregiver(s) able to verbalize/demonstrate skills taught by RN

10. Potential discharge plans for this patient

Nursing home placement for continued care
Discharge to home with home nursing services for
continued care
Symptom-controlled death with dignity in inpatient
setting
Discharge to home self-care

Decubitus Ulcer

1. Assessment of the patient problem

Obtain subjective data from the patient, family, or
caregiver(s)

2. Associated nursing diagnoses

Activity intolerance
Activity intolerance, high risk for
Body image disturbance
Constipation
Disuse syndrome, high risk for
Fatigue
Fear
Hopelessness
Infection, high risk for
Injury, high risk for
Mobility, impaired physical
Nutrition, altered: less than body requirements
Pain
Pain, chronic
Powerlessness
Role performance, altered
Self-care deficit, bathing/hygiene
Self-care deficit, dressing/grooming
Self-care deficit, feeding
Self-care deficit, toileting
Sensory/perceptual alterations (specify) (visual,
auditory, kinesthetic, gustatory, tactile, olfactory)
Sexuality patterns, altered
Skin integrity, impaired
Skin integrity, impaired, high risk for
Tissue integrity, impaired
Tissue perfusion, altered (specify type) (renal, cerebral,
cardiopulmonary, gastrointestinal, peripheral)
Trauma, high risk for

3. **Examples of objective data for documentation**
   Vital signs
   Decubitus ulcer description
   Tears, crying
   IV solution, rate ordered, site
   Presence of urinary or other catheter(s)
   Breath sounds
   Level of consciousness
   Vomiting
   Weight
   Lab or x-ray results
   Family/caregiver(s) with patient
   Intake and output
   Skin color
   Presence of impaction
   Restlessness
   Use of oxygen
   Position

4. **Examples of the assessment of the data**
   Unstable vital signs
   Alert, oriented x3
   Upset, depressed
   Patient in pain, uncomfortable
   IV infusing
   Patent urinary catheter
   Physician notified of noted change(s)
   Wound healing as evidenced by _____
   Impaction; unable to evacuate stool

5. **Examples of potential medical problems for this patient**
   Wound infection
   Cellulitis
   Osteomyelitis
   Tissue necrosis
   Chronic ulcers
   Other infection
   Trauma (falls)
   Immobility

6. **Examples of the documentation of potential nursing interventions/actions**

Comprehensive patient wound assessment completed
Patient monitored for signs, symptoms of infection
Venipuncture obtained as ordered
IV sites assessed for redness, other signs of infiltration
Wound site(s) cultured
Patient taught about new antibiotic regimen
Dressing changed per orders
IV solution of _____ started
Hydration/nutritional status assessed
Patient offered foods/beverages from lists of favorites provided by family
Taught family/caregiver(s) prescribed wound care, dressing procedures
Comfort measures provided
Support hose applied
Family conference held to determine how they can assist patient
Changed urinary catheter #_____, _____cc per physician order(s)
Checked for impaction per physician order(s)
Patient's position changed
Patient placed on air-fluidized therapy bed per physician order(s)
Patient medicated with pain medication prior to debridement
Enterostome nurse therapist consulted regarding wound care

7. **Examples of the evaluations of the interventions/actions**

Negative cultures
Blood tests (e.g., WBC) within normal range for patient
Afebrile
No evidence of impaction
Abdomen no longer distended
Vital signs within normal range for patient
Urinary output within normal range for patient

Temperature rechecked; now _____
Pain controlled as evidenced by _____
Pain relief expressed after administration of analgesic
Patient not vomiting after administration of antiemetic
suppository
Family/caregiver(s) demonstrated correct
procedure(s) as taught by RN
New granulation noted around perimeter of wound

8. **Other services that may be indicated and their
    associated interventions and goals/outcomes**

    Nurse aide

    Personal care
    ADL assistance
    Other duties
    Goals:
    >   Effective personal care provided
    >   Patient verbalizes comfort, feeling of well-being
    >   Assistance with ADL provided

    Physical therapy

    Evaluation
    Therapeutic exercise regimen
    Bed mobility exercises as tolerated
    Proper positioning
    ROM
    Active-assistive exercises
    Passive and active exercises
    Teach maintenance program
    Teach use of assistive devices as indicated
    Teach safe transfer techniques
    Chest physical therapy
    Goals:
    >   Increased mobility
    >   Patient able to use assistive devices
    >   Family or caregiver demonstrates safe transfer
    >   techniques
    >   Family/caregiver(s) able to demonstrate exercise
    >   regimen

Occupational therapy

Evaluation
ADL training
Upper extremity exercise and activity
Joint protection and functional positioning
Splints and orthoses
Goals:
> Functional mobility
> Increased quality of life
> Joints protected and in functional positioning

Chaplaincy

Spiritual support offered to patient,
family/caregiver(s)
Goals:
> Spiritual support provided to patient,
> family/caregiver(s)
> Referral to community spiritual resource(s) as
> indicated

Social work

Assessment of emotional/social factors
Financial resource information to patient,
family/caregiver(s)
Personal emergency response system referral where
appropriate
Goals:
> Problem identification and referral(s) to
> appropriate resources
> Patient discharged to appropriate level of care
> setting

Discharge planning nurse/team

Comprehensive patient evaluation
Communication of evaluation with other team
members, patient, family/caregiver(s)
Referral(s) to community resources
Goals:
> Referral information communicated to nurse in
> other setting

Meeting with patient/family to obtain agreement
on tentative plan

9. **Nursing goals and outcomes**

Daily implementation of care plan, created within
_____ hours of admission and updated and/or
reevaluated q _____ hours or as indicated by patient's
condition

Return to self-care or status prior to hospitalization,
pain-free with functional mobility and ambulation

Wound healing

Adequate hydration/nutritional status for healing

Infection-free wound site

Pain control

Patient/family/caregiver(s) taught and able to care for
patient

Compliance with regimens demonstrated by
patient/family in inpatient facility

10. **Potential discharge plans for this patient**

Nursing home placement

Discharge to home with caregiver(s) trained and able
to care for patient

Symptoms controlled until death

Discharge to home with home nursing services to
follow up on care plan

Diabetes Mellitus

1. Assessment of the patient problem

Obtain subjective data from the patient, family, or caregiver(s)

2. Associated nursing diagnoses

Activity intolerance
Activity intolerance, high risk for
Adjustment, impaired
Anxiety
Body image disturbance
Body temperature, altered, high risk for
Coping, ineffective family: compromised
Coping, ineffective family: disabling
Coping, ineffective individual
Denial, ineffective
Disuse syndrome, high risk for
Family processes, altered
Fatigue
Fear
Fluid volume deficit (1)
Fluid volume deficit, high risk for
Fluid volume excess
Gas exchange, impaired
Grieving, anticipatory
Grieving, dysfunctional
Hyperthermia
Hypothermia
Infection, high risk for
Injury, high risk for
Knowledge deficit (specify)
Mobility, impaired physical
Noncompliance (specify)
Nutrition, altered: high risk for more than body requirements
Nutrition, altered: less than body requirements

Nutrition, altered: more than body requirements
Pain
Pain, chronic
Sensory/perceptual alterations (specify) (visual, auditory, kinesthetic, gustatory, tactile, olfactory)
Sexual dysfunction
Sexuality patterns, altered
Skin integrity, impaired
Skin integrity, impaired, high risk for
Spiritual distress (distress of the human spirit)
Thought processes, altered
Tissue integrity, impaired
Tissue perfusion, altered (specify type) (renal, cerebral, cardiopulmonary, gastrointestinal, peripheral)
Trauma, high risk for
Unilateral neglect
Urinary elimination, altered patterns

3. **Examples of objective data for documentation**
   Vital signs
   Level of consciousness
   Slurred speech
   Tears, crying
   Hemiparesis
   Blood glucose levels
   Urine glucose
   Asymmetry in facial features
   Urinary catheter presence
   Lung sounds
   Weight
   Oxygen use
   Intake and output
   Skin color
   Acetone presence
   Impotence

4. **Examples of the assessment of the data**
   Unstable vital signs (e.g., BP high or low, febrile, change in vital signs)

Upset, depressed
IV infusing
Patent urinary catheter
Change in lung sounds
High blood pressure
Hyperglycemia
Hypoglycemia
Diabetic ketoacidosis

5. **Examples of potential medical problems for this patient**

Urinary tract infection
Pneumonia or other process
Peripheral vascular disease
Leg or foot ulcers
Hyperglycemia
Hypoglycemia
Arterial occlusive disease
Gangrene
Cellulitis
Hypertension
Neuropathy
Diabetic retinopathy
Ketoacidosis
Amputation
Angina, other cardiac pathology
Vasculitis
Monilial or other infections
Local tissue atrophy
Sexual dysfunction

6. **Examples of the documentation of potential nursing interventions/actions**

Assessed patient's baseline knowledge regarding aspects of care
Vital signs (specify routes) being measured q _____
Evaluated level of consciousness
Emotional support provided to patient and family
Taught medication regimen
Support hose applied

Taught signs, symptoms of
hyperglycemia/hypoglycemia
Taught patient to measure, record, and report blood
sugar(s)
Auscultation performed for respiratory
baseline/changes
Foot care regimen implemented
Daily weights
Patient and caregiver taught to mix insulins
Observed for potential infection at wound site
Assessed for amount, site(s) of fluid retention
Diet of _____ taught to patient and caregiver
Administered _____ units of _____ insulin sc
Taught patient and caregiver to draw up and
administer insulin
Teaching begun regarding diabetes management
regimen per facility protocol(s)
Taught importance of diet and eating at regular times
Blood glucose being monitored q _____; call physician
if over _____ or less than _____
Taught survival skills/emergency measures to patient
and family regarding hyperglycemia/hypoglycemia
Assessed and identified need for podiatry evaluation
Taught actions of ordered insulin(s)
Monitored pedal pulses
Taught urine testing for glucose/acetone
Taught safety measures regarding decreased sensation
(e.g., to avoid heating pads)

7. **Examples of the evaluations of the
   interventions/actions**

   Blood glucose _____, within normal range for patient
   Temperature rechecked at _____ PM; now _____,
   within normal range
   Pain controlled as evidenced by _____
   Caregiver demonstrated correct procedure of
   _____ as taught by RN
   Observed no evidence of infection at site; no heat,
   redness, swelling, drainage, or increased temperature
   noted

8. **Other services that may be indicated and their associated interventions and goals/outcomes**

   Nurse aide

   Personal care
   ADL assistance
   Other duties
   Goals:
   > Effective personal care provided
   > Assisted with ADL

   Chaplaincy

   Spiritual support offered to patient,
   family/caregiver(s)
   Goals:
   > Spiritual support provided to patient,
   > family/caregiver(s)

   Social work

   Assessment of social and emotional factors
   Counseling
   Financial assistance
   Arrangements for meal delivery program
   Goals:
   > Resources identified and referral(s) made to
   > community programs

   Discharge planning nurse/team

   Comprehensive evaluation of patient's needs
   Home nursing care referral
   Personal emergency response system referral
   Goals:
   > Patient and family ready for discharge

9. **Nursing goals and outcomes**

   Daily implementation of care plan, created within
   _____ hours of admission and updated and/or
   reevaluated q _____ hours or as indicated by patient's
   condition
   Return to self-care or status prior to hospitalization,

pain-free with functional mobility and ambulation
Diabetes mellitus controlled as evidenced by blood
glucose within normal range for patient
Patient/family taught regarding insulin or other
medications, diet regimens, and emergency measures

10. **Discharge plans for this patient**

Discharge to home; goals achieved
Nursing home placement
Discharge to home with home nursing services

Fracture Care (Orthopedic Care, Lower Extremity, Hip)

◆

1. **Assessment of the patient problem**
   Obtain subjective data from the patient, family, or caregiver(s)

2. **Associated nursing diagnoses**
   Activity intolerance
   Anxiety
   Constipation
   Disuse syndrome, high risk for
   Fear
   Infection, high risk for
   Injury, high risk for
   Mobility, impaired physical
   Pain
   Pain, chronic
   Role performance, altered
   Self-care deficit, bathing/hygiene
   Self-care deficit, dressing/grooming
   Self-care deficit, feeding
   Self-care deficit, toileting
   Sexuality patterns, altered
   Skin integrity, impaired
   Skin integrity, impaired, high risk for
   Sleep pattern disturbance
   Tissue perfusion, altered (peripheral)
   Urinary elimination, altered patterns

3. **Examples of objective data for documentation**
   Vital signs
   Bleeding
   Vomiting
   Sweating
   Restlessness

IV solution, rate ordered, site description
Urinary catheter, color, amount, odor
Lung sounds
Traction, cast, position

4. **Examples of the assessment of the data**
Unstable vital signs (e.g., BP high or low, febrile, change in vital signs)
Postoperative wound site bleeding
Pain
IV infusing
Patent urinary catheter
Change in lung sounds
Traction in place at _____lbs
No swelling or redness at cast site

5. **Examples of potential medical problems for this patient**
Urinary tract infection
Pneumonia or other lung process
Operative wound site infection
Thrombophlebitis
Fat embolism

6. **Examples of the documentation of potential nursing interventions/actions**
BP, pulse, respirations, temperature (specify route) being measured q _____
Bleeding amount being monitored q _____; report findings to physician
Administered antiemetic medication IM q _____ per physician order(s)
Administered pain relief medication q _____ per physician order(s)
Changed or started IV solution of _____, _____ cc per _____ hour
Obtained urine specimen for UA/C & S per physician order(s)

Venipuncture obtained for monitoring anticoagulant q
_____

Taught regarding medications and side effects
Assessed hydration/nutritional status
Assessed lung, cardiovascular status
Laxative of patient's choice (_____) administered
per order
Changed catheter #_____, _____ cc per physician
order(s)
Patient reminded to cough and deep breathe q_____
Repositioned patient into _____ position with
traction at _____

7. **Examples of the evaluations of the
   interventions/actions**

   Temperature rechecked at _____ PM; now _____
   No vomiting; patient reports no nausea
   Patient verbalizes pain relief; no longer restless
   Patient states that nausea accompanies pain; has no
   relief from nausea or pain
   IV patent; site without problems
   Catheter patent; yellow urine draining into drainage
   bag
   Patient coughing and deep breathing as instructed;
   lungs clear
   Patient expresses comfort after repositioning

8. **Other services that may be indicated and their
   associated interventions and goals/outcomes**

   Nurse aide

   Personal care
   ADL assistance
   Other duties
   Goals:
   > Patient clean and comfortable
   > Effective personal hygiene

Physical therapy

Evaluation
Therapeutic exercise regimen; transfer training or techniques
Progressive gait training with assistive device
Chest physiotherapy
Ultrasound
ADL training
Strengthening exercises
Progressive/resistive exercises
Bed mobility and trapeze
Passive and active exercises
Crutch walking
Transfer or mobility skills
Goals:
> Patient using safety skills taught and assistive device(s)
> Functional ambulation

Occupational therapy

Evaluation
ADL training program
Increase upper extremity strength through exercises and activities
Other ADL training as indicated
Teach alternative bathing, dressing, feeding skills
Goals:
> Functional mobility
> Increased strength
> Maximum function

Chaplaincy

Spiritual support offered to patient, family/caregiver(s)
Support to elderly spouse or caregiver
Goals:
> Spiritual support provided to patient, family/caregiver(s)

Social work

Assessment of social and emotional factors
Counseling
Financial assistance
Nursing home placement assistance
Arrange for meal program(s)
Goals:
> Resources identified and referral(s) made to
> community programs

Discharge planning nurse/team

Home nursing care referral
Personal emergency response system referral
Goals:
> Patient and family ready for discharge

9. **Nursing goals and outcomes**

   Daily implementation of care plan, created within
   _____ hours of admission and updated and/or
   reevaluated q _____ hours or as indicated by patient's
   condition
   Return to self-care or status prior to hospitalization,
   pain-free with functional mobility and ambulation

10. **Potential discharge plans for this patient**

    Discharge to home; goals achieved
    Nursing home placement
    Discharge to home with follow-up therapy in home
    setting

Hypertension

1. **Assessment of the patient problem**
   Obtain subjective data from the patient, family, or
   caregiver(s)

2. **Associated nursing diagnoses**
   Anxiety
   Cardiac output, decreased
   Injury, high risk for
   Knowledge deficit (specify)
   Noncompliance (specify)
   Nutrition, altered: more than body requirements
   Pain
   Powerlessness

3. **Examples of objective data for documentation**
   Level of consciousness
   Blood pressure readings
   Medications taken by patient
   Weight
   ECG, other diagnostic results
   History of seizures, faintness, blurred vision

4. **Examples of the assessment of the data**
   High blood pressure
   Overweight or obesity
   Headache, blurred vision

5. **Examples of potential medical problems for this
   patient**
   CVA
   Renal disease
   Blindness
   AMI
   TIA
   Other system processes

6. **Examples of the documentation of potential nursing interventions/actions**

Venipunctures obtained as ordered
Comprehensive nursing assessment completed on admission
Intake and output being monitored
Emotional support provided to patient and family
Checked blood pressure in both arms: sitting, lying, and standing
Assessed for postural changes in blood pressure readings
Administered ordered antihypertensive medications
Physician notified of change in blood pressure readings

7. **Examples of the evaluations of the interventions/actions**

Patient diuresing
Patient has weight loss of _____ since (specify date)
Blood pressure decreased to _____, within normal range for patient
Patient maintaining ordered bed rest
IV patent and maintenance fluid infusing at ordered rate

8. **Other services that may be indicated and their associated interventions and goals/outcomes**

Nurse aide

Personal care
ADL assistance
Other duties
Goals:
   Effective personal care provided
   Patient clean and comfortable

Chaplaincy

Spiritual support offered to patient, family/caregiver(s)

Goals:

> Spiritual support provided to patient, family/caregiver(s)
> Referral to community spiritual resource(s) as indicated

Social work

Assessment of emotional/social factors impacting on health

Financial assistance

Referral(s) to identified community resources

Goals:

> Resources identified and referral(s) completed

Discharge planning nurse/team

Evaluation of patient's needs

Home nursing care referral where appropriate

Goals:

> Patient referred to home nursing service for follow-up per physician order(s)
> Family and patient notified of plan prior to discharge

9. **Nursing goals and outcomes**

   Daily implementation of care plan, created within _____ hours of admission and updated and/or reevaluated q _____ hours or as indicated by patient's condition

   Return to self-care or status prior to hospitalization, pain-free with functional mobility and ambulation

   Teaching understood and integrated into daily living

   Blood pressure controlled

   Adherence to medication, diet, exercise regimens

10. **Potential discharge plans for this patient**

    Discharge to home; self-care

    Discharge to home with skilled support of community home nursing program

Impaction

1. **Assessment of the patient problem**

   Obtain subjective data from the patient, family, or caregiver(s)

2. **Associated nursing diagnoses**

   Constipation
   Constipation, colonic
   Constipation, perceived
   Fluid volume deficit
   Fluid volume deficit, high risk for
   Pain
   Pain, chronic
   Self-care deficit, toileting

3. **Examples of objective data for documentation**

   Hard (or soft) stool in rectum
   Date of last bowel movement (specify date)
   Stomach distended or distention
   Impaction removed
   Abdominal tenderness
   Suppository insertion
   Poor hydration/nutritional status
   History of hospitalization; change in usual level of activity
   Hemorrhoids

4. **Examples of the assessment of the data**

   Unable to evacuate stool
   Abdominal distention
   Laxative dependence
   Pain
   Impaction present
   Upset, uncomfortable

5. **Examples of potential medical problems for this patient**

Rectal fissure
Perforation
Immobility (as hospitalization continues)
Dehydration
Nausea, vomiting

6. **Examples of the documentation of potential nursing interventions/actions**

Evaluated for and removed impaction per physician order(s)
Obtained a nursing history of prior problems/habits
Implemented a hydration schedule
Dietary instruction on appropriate diet initiated for patient
Implemented bowel regimen to prevent further constipation
Taught patient, family/caregiver(s) bowel regimen and diet
Assessed hydration/nutritional status
Taught regarding increase in fiber, fruit, and fluid diet
Administered enema per physician order(s)
Taught suppository administration

7. **Examples of the evaluations of the interventions/actions**

Checked for impaction; digital exam showed

_____

New bowel regimen effective: patient having bowel movements every other day (will continue regimen)
Abdomen no longer distended
Patient verbalized relief of pain, discomfort, distention after enema

8. **Other services that may be indicated and their associated interventions and goals/outcomes**

    Nurse aide

    Personal care
    ADL assistance
    Encourage/offer patient fluids every hour and chart intake by cc
    Goals:
    >   Effective personal hygiene/personal care provided
    >   Patient clean and comfortable

9. **Nursing goals and outcomes**

    Daily implementation of care plan, created within _____ hours of admission and updated and/or reevaluated q _____ hours or as indicated by patient's condition
    Return to self-care or status prior to hospitalization, pain-free with functional mobility and ambulation
    Daily compliance with increased fluid, fiber, fruit dietary regimen as tolerated
    Bowel movements occurring
    Patient without initial complaint of discomfort; no longer impacted; beginning new diet/fluid/exercise regimen as appropriate
    Dietary changes integrated into daily lifestyle

10. **Potential discharge plans for this patient**

    Discharge to home without impaction and with patient and/or family/caregiver(s) instructed on new diet and bowel regimens

Intravenous Therapy Care

◆

1. **Assessment of the patient problem**
   Obtain subjective data from the patient, family, or caregiver(s)

2. **Associated nursing diagnoses**
   Anxiety
   Fear
   Fluid volume deficit
   Fluid volume deficit, high risk for
   Fluid volume excess
   Infection, high risk for
   Pain
   Skin integrity, impaired
   Skin integrity, impaired, high risk for

3. **Examples of objective data for documentation**
   Vital signs
   IV fluid composition
   Rate of ordered infusion
   Additives
   Specific site of IV
   Weight
   Intake and output
   Swelling, redness at IV site
   Skin turgor
   Lab values (e.g., serum BUN, Na, K)
   Patient in for 6 weeks of antibiotic therapy
   Moist rales

4. **Examples of the assessment of the data**
   Weight less than yesterday, or other specified date
   IV infusing
   Patient diuresing
   Infiltrated IV site

Pain at IV site
Physician notified of change identified

5. **Examples of potential medical problems for this patient**
   Fluid overload
   CHF/pulmonary edema
   Infected IV site
   Cellulitis
   Electrolyte imbalances
   Phlebitis
   Other local or systemic infections
   Air emboli
   Infiltration
   Thrombosis

6. **Examples of the documentation of potential nursing interventions/actions**
   IV site assessed for signs of infection: redness, tenderness, warmth, and/or swelling
   RN explained procedure of starting IV to patient and family
   Patient taught to not move arm site excessively because of risk of moving/dislodging catheter, causing infiltration at site
   Nurse explained infusion pump to patient
   RN cautioned patient to report any pain, tenderness, or swelling
   Angiocatheter removed by RN; no swelling, redness, or tenderness noted
   IV infusion dressing site changed per facility protocol

7. **Examples of the evaluations of the interventions/actions**
   IV is patent and infusing as ordered
   Observed no evidence of infection at site; without heat, redness, swelling, or tenderness

Urinary output within normal range for patient
Patient resting comfortably after site change and
backrub

8. **Other services that may be indicated and their
   associated interventions and goals/outcomes**

   Nurse aide

   Personal care
   ADL assistance
   Other duties
   Goals:
   > Effective personal care provided
   > Patient clean and comfortable

   Chaplaincy

   Spiritual support offered to patient,
   family/caregiver(s)
   Goals:
   > Spiritual support provided to patient,
   > family/caregiver(s)
   > Referral to community spiritual resource(s) as
   > indicated

   Social work

   Assessment of emotional/social factors impacting on
   health
   Financial resource information to patient,
   family/caregiver(s)
   Goals:
   > Problem identification and referral(s) to resources

   Discharge planning nurse/team

   Comprehensive patient evaluation
   Referral(s) to community health resources
   Goals:
   > Comprehensive predischarge evaluation
   > Referral(s) to community home nursing program
   > for follow-up care

9. **Nursing goals and outcomes**

Daily implementation of care plan, created within
_____ hours of admission and updated and/or
reevaluated q _____ hours or as indicated by patient's
condition
Return to self-care or status prior to hospitalization,
pain-free with functional mobility and ambulation
Adequate hydration
IV antibiotic therapy
Infection-free at sites
Patient returned to self-care status

10. **Potential discharge plans for this patient**

Discharge to home; self-care without IV
Discharge to home with IV and referral to home
nursing service for follow-up care

Mastectomy Care

◆

1. **Assessment of the patient problem**

   Obtain subjective data from the patient, family, or caregiver(s)

2. **Associated nursing diagnoses**

   Activity intolerance
   Activity intolerance, high risk for
   Adjustment, impaired
   Anxiety
   Body image disturbance
   Decisional conflict (e.g., treatment)
   Family processes, altered
   Fatigue
   Fear
   Grieving, anticipatory
   Pain
   Self-care deficit, bathing/hygiene
   Self-care deficit, dressing/grooming
   Sexuality patterns, altered
   Skin integrity, impaired
   Skin integrity, impaired, high risk for
   Tissue integrity, impaired

3. **Examples of objective data for documentation**

   Site of breast lump or mass
   History of prior related surgeries (dates)
   Vital signs
   Presence of visitors
   Weight
   Lab results
   Wound dressing postoperatively
   Level of consciousness

4. **Examples of the assessment of the data**
    Unstable vital signs
    Weight loss
    Pain, other symptoms
    Febrile
    Physician notified or change identified

5. **Examples of potential medical problems for this patient**
    Wound infection
    Lymphedema
    Dehiscence
    Hemorrhage
    Progression/complications from the original pathology (cancer) necessitating the mastectomy

6. **Examples of the documentation of potential nursing interventions/actions**
    Comprehensive preoperative nursing assessment completed
    RN conducted preoperative teaching with patient/family
    Teaching included role of family in care
    Patient taught importance of deep breathing and coughing postoperatively
    Postoperative assessment of patient on return to unit completed
    Pain, nausea, other symptoms evaluated and reported
    Emotional support provided to patient and family
    Comfort measure of backrub provided to patient
    Physician notified of change in patient's condition (specify)
    Patient observed for signs, symptoms of infection postoperatively
    Evaluated postoperative wound site and drains
    Administered analgesic as ordered

Psychosocial assessment of patient/family performed regarding disease/prognosis

Pain evaluation done, including site(s), duration, characteristics, relief measures

Assisted patient with progressive muscle relaxation, other measures to assist in control of anxiety and/or pain relief

Incision site/dressing checked for bleeding

Affected arm elevated after care of dressing/drainage system

Nurse listened to patient's feelings about her loss and concerns

Affected arm checked for swelling, circulatory problems

Patient taught to watch for and report any redness, swelling, warmth, drainage, or odor on return home

Patient taught about need to protect affected arm from injury or infection

Listened to patient's concerns after pathology report and subsequent treatment course was discussed with her by physician

7. **Examples of the evaluations of the intervention/actions**

Pain relief expressed after administration of ordered analgesic

Lab value of _____, within normal range for patient

Family/caregiver(s) demonstrated correct procedure as taught by RN

Unexpected amount of bloody drainage noted— physician notified

Patient able to void without problem after catheter removed

Successful plan as evidenced by _____

Drainage in closed self-suction drain decreasing to _____

Patient progressively learning wound site care

8. **Other services that may be indicated and their associated interventions and goals/outcomes**

Nurse aide

Personal care
ADL assistance
Other duties
Goals:
> Effective personal care provided
> Patient clean and comfortable

Physical therapy

Evaluation
Passive, active, active-assistive exercises
ADL assessment preoperatively and postoperatively
Home exercise program
Pain assessment/reduction measures
Goals:
> Knowledge of home exercise regimen by discharge
> Function maintained
> Severity of pain decreased

Chaplaincy

Spiritual support offered to patient,
family/caregiver(s)
Goals:
> Spiritual support provided to patient,
> family/caregiver(s)
> Referral to community spiritual resource(s) as
> indicated

Social work

Assessment of social and emotional factors impacting
on health
Financial resource information to patient,
family/caregiver(s)
Referral(s) to identified community resources
Goals:
> Problem identification and referral(s) to resources
> for follow-up
> Patient/family notified of plan prior to discharge

Discharge planning nurse/team

Comprehensive patient evaluation
Communication of identified needs to team members
Referral(s) to community resources
Goals:
> Home nursing care referral completed where appropriate
> Patient referred to "Reach for Recovery" program
> Referral to community physical rehabilitation program for postmastectomy patients

9. **Nursing goals and outcomes**

   Daily implementation of care plan, created within _____ hours of admission and updated and/or reevaluated q _____ hours or as indicated by patient's condition
   Return to self-care or status prior to hospitalization, pain-free with functional mobility and ambulation
   Pain-free
   Ambulatory or presurgery mobility status
   Self-care and able to do exercises taught by RN
   Afebrile; wound site infection-free
   Patient able to care for wound site independently
   Patient able to do self-exam on breast
   Patient adapting to diagnosis/prognosis and follow-up needed

10. **Potential discharge plans for this patient**

    Discharge to home; self-care
    Discharge to home with community home nursing services follow-up

Osteoarthritis

1. **Assessment of the patient problem**
   Obtain subjective data from the patient, family, or
   caregiver(s)

2. **Associated nursing diagnoses**
   Activity intolerance
   Activity intolerance, high risk for
   Body image disturbance
   Disuse syndrome, high risk for
   Fatigue
   Fear
   Hopelessness
   Infection, high risk for
   Injury, high risk for
   Knowledge deficit (specify)
   Mobility, impaired physical
   Noncompliance (specify)
   Pain
   Pain, chronic
   Powerlessness
   Self-care deficit, bathing/hygiene
   Self-care deficit, dressing/grooming
   Self-care deficit, feeding
   Self-care deficit, toileting
   Role performance, altered
   Sleep pattern disturbance
   Spiritual distress (distress of the human spirit)
   Trauma, high risk for
   Urinary retention

3. **Examples of objective data for documentation**
   Vital signs
   Results of lab data/serological studies (e.g., uric acid,
   erythrocyte sedimentation rate)

Medications that patient takes at home
Morning stiffness
Swelling in affected joint(s)
Weight loss
Warm, tender joints
Joint deformity
Presence of family/caregiver(s)

4. **Examples of the assessment of the data**

   Inflammation present in joint(s)
   Febrile
   Weight loss
   Limited ROM
   Uncontrolled pain

5. **Examples of potential medical problems for this patient**

   Hypertension
   Surgeries (e.g., joint replacement, osteotomy)
   Major organ systems involvement
   Side effects of multiple drug therapies

6. **Examples of the documentation of potential nursing interventions/actions**

   Comprehensive pain assessment and regimen implemented
   Administered gold therapy injection
   Comfort measures provided, specifically back massage
   Taught patient and family correct body alignment, posture, and positioning
   Taught patient and family about arthritis and care
   Taught patient progressive muscle relaxation techniques
   Patient repositioned to prevent joint deformity
   Warm bath given to patient this AM
   Patient monitored for untoward effects of steroid therapy

7. **Examples of the evaluations of the interventions/actions**

Patient verbalizes pain relief
Patient can relax (relaxing) muscles
Afebrile
Joints now without heat, pain, or swelling
Patient can verbalize and/or demonstrate what RN has taught
Patient has more stamina than on admission; can walk 10 ft with assistance
Patient now having uninterrupted periods of sleep
Patient has incorporated teaching into daily routine
Early morning stiffness relieved after baths

8. **Other services that may be indicated and their associated interventions and goals/outcomes**

Nurse aide

Personal care
ADL assistance
Other duties
Goals:
    Effective personal care provided
    Patient clean and comfortable

Physical therapy

Evaluation
Therapeutic exercise regimen
ROM
Bed mobility exercises as tolerated
Strengthening exercises
Teach use of assistive devices as indicated
Paraffin treatments
Moist warm heat applications
Applications of cold alternating with heat therapy
Therapeutic massage
Teach proper use (or avoidance of) heat modalities during acute inflammation, and as inflammation subsides and there is chronic pain
Whirlpool therapy

Teach principles of joint protection (especially during periods of joint inflammation)
Reduce joint activity when indicated
Goals:
>Joint mobility maintained
>Patient able to use assistive devices effectively
>Home exercise regimen taught to family
>Increased mobility since admission
>Prevention of further complications, deformity

Occupational therapy

Evaluation
ADL assessment and training
Upper extremity therapeutic exercises and activities
Teach conservation-of-energy techniques
Evaluation of need for splints and application of splints
Joint protection and functional positioning
Teach use of assistive devices
Splints and orthoses for upper extremities
Goals:
>Splinting aids in use to maintain joint function
>Increased coordination, strength in ADL
>Patient using conservation-of-energy techniques taught
>Patient using ADL assistive devices

Chaplaincy

Spiritual support offered to patient, family/caregiver(s)
Goals:
>Spiritual support provided to patient, family/caregiver(s)
>Referral to community spiritual resource(s) as indicated

Social work

Assessment of emotional/social factors
Identification of financial resources
Personal emergency response system referral where appropriate

Goals:
> Problem identification and referral(s) to appropriate community resources, including information about support groups

Discharge planning nurse/team
Comprehensive patient evaluation
Communication of identified needs with other team members and patient, family/caregiver(s)
Referral(s) to community resources
Goals:
> Referral information communicated to nurse in the facility or agency that patient is referred to for follow-up care

9. **Nursing goals and outcomes**

   Daily implementation of care plan, created within _____ hours of admission and updated and/or reevaluated q _____ hours or as indicated by patient's condition
   Return to self-care or status prior to hospitalization, pain-free with functional mobility and ambulation
   Pain relief
   Swelling, inflammation decreased since admission
   Afebrile
   Patient or family/caregiver(s) able to verbalize and demonstrate skills for patient's care as taught by RN
   Patient able to use assistive devices safely and effectively

10. **Potential discharge plans for this patient**

    Nursing home placement
    Discharge to home with patient returned to previous level of functioning
    Referral to home nursing agency

Ostomy

1. **Assessment of the patient problem**

   Obtain subjective data from the patient, family, or caregiver(s)

2. **Associated nursing diagnoses**

   Anxiety
   Body image disturbance
   Bowel incontinence
   Fatigue
   Fear
   Fluid volume deficit, high risk for
   Grieving, anticipatory
   Knowledge deficit (specify)
   Nutrition, altered: high risk for more than body requirements
   Nutrition, altered: less than body requirements
   Nutrition, altered: more than body requirements
   Pain
   Role performance, altered
   Self-care deficit, toileting
   Sexuality patterns, altered
   Skin integrity, impaired
   Skin integrity, impaired, high risk for
   Self-esteem disturbance
   Urinary elimination, altered patterns

3. **Examples of objective data for documentation**

   Leaking appliance/odor
   Vital signs
   Description of ostomy
   Type of ostomy appliance in use
   Type of ostomy (single- or double-barreled colostomy, ileoconduit, ileostomy)
   Description of effluent
   Weight

Dietary information
Lab or x-ray results
Bleeding from ostomy site
Nausea and/or vomiting
Amount of output from ostomy
Breakdown of skin integrity

4. **Examples of the assessment of the data**

Weight loss
Abdominal (or other) pain
Change in patient's condition noted; physician notified
Peristomal skin excoriation; enterostomy therapy (ET) nurse contacted
Caregiver unable to provide ostomy care required
Possible allergy to sealant/appliances used

5. **Examples of potential medical problems for this patient**

Stenosis
Retracted stoma
Prolapse
Necrosis
Perforation
Hernia
Obstruction
Hemorrhage
Infection

6. **Examples of the documentation of potential nursing interventions/actions**

Comprehensive baseline patient assessment completed on admission
ET nurse consulted prior to surgery, where possible—communicates to surgeon findings and site selected for stoma and marks patient's abdomen
Skin prep procedures completed per physician order(s)
Preoperative teaching by ET nurse completed with patient, family/caregiver(s)

Emotional support provided to patient and family with new diagnosis of cancer

Postoperative wound assessment completed

ET nurse in to meet with patient and family regarding new ostomy

RN listened to patient's concerns about sexuality with ostomy

Trained ostomy volunteer from community in to visit patient

Skin integrity being assessed every dressing/site change

Teaching continued regarding self-care at home

Patient taught to be prepared for "accidents"; to carry small bag with supplies, including one of each appliance used and a small plastic bag for disposal

Patient taught regarding importance of specific skin care regimen ordered

Patient taught modification of appliance to ensure fit

Dietary teaching started, with specific foods to avoid

Assessed output for color, frequency, amount

Stoma site cleansed and cared for per physician order(s) (specify)

RN administered ordered analgesic

Daily weights obtained

NG tube residual gastric content measured

7. **Examples of the evaluations of the interventions/actions**

Pain relief expressed after administration of ordered analgesic

Patient/caregiver demonstrated correct procedure as taught by RN

Weight of _____ is a decrease of _____ lb since (specify date)

IV antibiotic hung and infused without untoward reaction

Patient correctly demonstrated skills taught by RN

Patient able to rest after backrub and administration of analgesic

Patient ambulating in hall without assistance
Patient is deep breathing and coughing as taught
Patient able to perform skin care and appliance
application
Stoma/wound site healing occurring

8. **Other services that may be indicated and their associated interventions and goals/outcomes**

Nurse aide

Personal care
ADL assistance
Other duties
Goals:
> Effective personal care provided
> Patient is clean and comfortable

Enterostomal therapy nurse

Patient assessment
Teaching/training
Other consultative or clinical services based on
patient/family needs
Goals:
> Patient/caregiver able to provide adequate care
> Problem areas identified and will be followed up
> on outpatient basis
> Patient starting integration of new body image

Chaplaincy

Spiritual support offered to patient,
family/caregiver(s) (e.g., in patient with new or
chronic diagnosis of cancer and associated body image
changes)
Goals:
> Spiritual support provided to patient,
> family/caregiver(s)
> Referral to community spiritual resource(s) as
> indicated

Social work

Assessment of social/emotional factors
Financial resource information (e.g., needed supplies)
Referral(s) to identified community resources
Goals:
>   Problem identification and referral(s) to resources
>   Communication with patient, family to
>   communicate plan prior to discharge

Discharge planning nurse/team

Comprehensive patient evaluation
Communication of needs with team members
Referral(s) to community health resources
Goals:
>   Home nursing care referral accomplished;
>   communication with nurse in home nursing
>   program who will follow-up with patient and
>   family in patient's home

Hospice or home care referral per physician order(s)

9. **Nursing goals and outcomes**

    Daily implementation of care plan, created within
    _____ hours of admission and updated and/or
    reevaluated q _____ hours or as indicated by patient's
    condition
    Return to self-care or status prior to hospitalization,
    pain-free with functional mobility and ambulation
    Patient adapting to altered body image
    Patient/family able to care for ostomy on daily basis
    Patient has phone number of community support
    group
    Infection-free, healing site(s)
    Hydration/nutritional status adequate
    Elimination within normal for patient range
    Proper-fitting appliance

10. **Potential discharge plans for this patient**
    Discharge to home; self-care
    Discharge to home with support and skilled follow-up
    by nurses in the community
    Nursing home placement due to other problems and
    level of care needed
    Comfortable, symptom-controlled death in inpatient
    facility

Peripheral Vascular Disease

◆

1. **Assessment of the patient problem**

   Obtain subjective data from the patient, family, or caregiver(s)

2. **Associated nursing diagnoses**

   Anxiety
   Body image disturbance
   Cardiac output, decreased
   Infection, high risk for
   Injury, high risk for
   Mobility, impaired physical
   Noncompliance (specify)
   Pain
   Pain, chronic
   Powerlessness
   Sensory/perceptual alterations (tactile)
   Sexuality patterns, altered
   Tissue integrity, impaired
   Tissue perfusion, altered (specify type) (renal, cerebral, cardiopulmonary, gastrointestinal, peripheral)
   Trauma, high risk for

3. **Examples of objective data for documentation**

   Vital signs
   Open wound site(s), location, description
   Weight
   Visitors/family accompanying patient
   Intake and output
   Oxygen use
   Presence of urinary or other catheter(s)
   Lab test results
   Patient position
   Swelling

4. **Examples of the assessment of the data**

   Unstable vital signs (e.g., BP high or low, febrile, change in vital signs)
   Upset, depressed, uncomfortable
   IV infusing
   Patent urinary catheter
   Alert, oriented x3
   Weight loss or gain
   Dyspnea
   Fatigue
   Physician notified of change _____
   Wound healing as evidenced by _____
   Pain relief after administration of ordered analgesic

5. **Examples of potential medical problems for this patient**

   Wound infection
   Cellulitis
   Tissue necrosis
   Chronic stasis ulcers
   Dermatitis
   Trauma
   Venous insufficiency

6. **Examples of the documentation of potential nursing interventions/actions**

   Comprehensive baseline nursing assessment completed
   Wound site(s) cultured
   Patient taught regarding new antibiotic regimen
   Administered first dose of new regimen _____
   Assessment of hydration/nutritional status completed
   Patient/family taught prescribed wound care; dressing procedures
   Cautioned patient to avoid standing for long periods of time

Cautioned patient to avoid wearing tight, restrictive clothes
Patient cautioned not to cross legs
Support hose applied
Comfort measures and analgesic administered to decrease pain
Provided and taught skin care of affected areas
Dressing removed
Dressing applied per facility protocol(s)
Patient medicated with analgesic prior to dressing change
Patient's affected lower leg and foot soaked in

_____

Taught safety measures regarding decreased sensation in lower extremities (e.g., avoid use of heating pads, electric blankets)
Venipuncture obtained
Physician notified of change in patient's condition
Exercises provided to increase circulation, decrease edema

7. **Examples of the evaluations of the interventions/actions**

Pain relief expressed after administration of pain medication
Decreased swelling noted in affected LLE
Measurement in leg decreased to _____
Healing, granulation noted in affected lower extremity
Skin now pink around perimeter of open site(s)
Pain controlled as evidenced by _____
Wound site now without swelling, redness, or exudate
Temperature rechecked; now at _____, within normal range for patient
Caregiver demonstrated correct procedure of dressing change
Negative cultures
WBC within normal range for patient

8. **Other services that may be indicated and their associated interventions and goals/outcomes**

Nurse aide

Personal care
ADL assistance
Other duties
Goals:
> Effective personal care provided
> Patient verbalizes comfort
> Assistance with ADL provided

Chaplaincy

Spiritual support offered to patient, family/caregiver(s)
Goals:
> Spiritual support provided to patient, family/caregiver(s)
> Referral to community spiritual resource(s) as indicated

Social work

Assessment of social and emotional factors
Counseling
Financial assistance
Referral(s) to resources as identified by needs assessment
Goals:
> Resources identified and referral(s) made to community programs

Discharge planning nurse/team

Comprehensive evaluation of patient's needs
Home nursing care referral
Goals:
> Patient and family prepared for discharge
> Patient discharged to appropriate level of care setting

9. **Nursing goals and outcomes**
    Daily implementation of care plan, created within
    _____ hours of admission and updated and/or
    reevaluated q _____ hours or as indicated by patient's
    condition
    Return to self-care or status prior to hospitalization,
    pain-free with functional mobility and ambulation
    Pain control
    Infection-free
    Patient compliance with regimen

10. **Potential discharge plans for this patient**
    Discharge to home; returned to prior self-care status
    Nursing home placement for continued care
    Discharge to home with home nursing services for
    continued care

Pneumonia

1. **Assessment of the patient problem**

   Obtain subjective data from the patient, family, or caregiver(s)

2. **Associated nursing diagnoses**

   Activity intolerance
   Activity intolerance, high risk for
   Airway clearance, ineffective
   Anxiety
   Aspiration, high risk for
   Body temperature, altered, high risk for
   Breathing pattern, ineffective
   Fatigue
   Fear
   Gas exchange, impaired
   Infection, high risk for
   Mobility, impaired physical
   Nutrition, altered: less than body requirements
   Pain
   Self-care deficit, bathing/hygiene
   Self-care deficit, dressing/grooming
   Self-care deficit, feeding
   Self-care deficit, toileting
   Sexuality patterns, altered
   Sleep pattern disturbance
   Swallowing, impaired

3. **Examples of objective data for documentation**

   Use of oxygen
   Results of chest x-ray
   Vital signs
   Rhonchi, rales
   Diaphoresis
   Cough
   Chills

Results of WBC, ABGs
Sputum production

4. **Examples of the assessment of the data**
   Positive cultures, gram stains
   Unstable vital signs (e.g., febrile)
   IV infusing
   Alert, oriented x3
   Change noted on breath sounds
   Upset, depressed
   Productive cough

5. **Examples of potential medical problems for this patient**
   Respiratory distress
   Relapse/recurring pneumonia
   Dehydration (nausea, vomiting, anorexia)
   Confusion
   Pleurisy
   Lung abscess
   Pulmonary edema
   Other system pathologies

6. **Examples of the documentation of potential nursing interventions/actions**
   Comprehensive baseline patient assessment performed
   Administered antibiotic(s) of _____
   Venipuncture obtained as ordered
   Taught patient/family/caregiver about use of oxygen
   Administered nebulizer therapy
   Evaluated hydration/nutritional status
   Vital signs being monitored q 2 hours
   Patient taught skills to cough/expectorate effectively
   Patient maintained in semi-Fowler's or upright position
   Treatment of chest physiotherapy/postural drainage provided
   Fluids of patient's choice being encouraged

Intake and output being monitored
IV site care provided per facility protocol
Urinary catheter care provided
Comfort measure of back massage provided
Administered ordered antipyretic
Tracheobronchial suctioning provided
Appropriate skills being taught to patient/family to assist in care

7. **Examples of the evaluations of the interventions/actions**

Pain relief expressed after administration of analgesic
ABGs now _____, within normal range for patient
Temperature now _____, within normal range for patient, after administration of antipyretic
Caregiver demonstrated correct procedure of _____ as taught by RN
Patient able to sleep after chest physical therapy session
Family able to demonstrate skills taught by RN
Patient able to rest between planned interventions/therapy sessions

8. **Other services that may be indicated and their associated interventions and goals/outcomes**

Nurse aide

Personal care
ADL assistance
Other duties
Goals:
> Effective personal care provided
> Patient clean and comfortable

Physical therapy

Evaluation
Chest physical therapy
Therapeutic exercise regimen
ROM
Bed mobility exercises as tolerated

Breathing exercises
Strengthening exercises
Teach use of assistive devices as indicated
Goals:
>   Pulmonary program goals achieved
>   Increased mobility
>   Discharged to prior mobility status
>   Patient, family/caregiver(s) able to demonstrate
>   home exercise regimen

Occupational therapy

Evaluation
Conservation-of-energy techniques
ADL training
Functional mobility
Goals:
>   Patient using conservation-of-energy techniques
>   Patient able to use ADL assistive devices

Speech-language pathology

Evaluation
Swallowing assessment if indicated
Goals:
>   Effective, safe swallowing

Chaplaincy

Spiritual support offered to patient,
family/caregiver(s)
Goals:
>   Spiritual support provided to patient,
>   family/caregiver(s)

Social work

Assessment of emotional/social factors impacting on
health
Financial resource information to patient,
family/caregiver(s)
Referral(s) to identified community resources
Goals:
>   Problem identification and referral(s) to
>   appropriate community resources

Personal emergency response system referral made, where appropriate

Discharge planning nurse/team
Comprehensive patient evaluation
Communication of evaluation with other team members, patient, family/caregiver(s)
Referral(s) to community resources
Goals:
Referral information communicated to nurse in facility or program that patient is transferring to
Meeting with patient, family/caregiver(s) to facilitate continuity of care

9. **Nursing goals and outcomes**
Daily implementation of care plan, created within _____ hours of admission and updated and/or reevaluated q _____ hours or as indicated by patient's condition
Return to self-care or status prior to hospitalization, pain-free with functional mobility and ambulation
Improved air exchange
Decreased subjective shortness of breath
Temperature within normal range for patient
Stable respiratory status
Adequate hydration/nutritional status
Patient, family/caregiver(s) demonstrates/verbalizes care of patient on discharge

10. **Potential discharge plans for this patient**
Nursing home placement for continued therapy, care
Discharge to home with caregiver(s) able to care for patient
Discharge to home with home nursing care services
Symptom-controlled death in inpatient setting

Sickle Cell Anemia

◆

1. **Assessment of the patient problem**

   Obtain subjective data from the patient, family, or caregiver(s)

2. **Associated nursing diagnoses**

   Body image disturbance
   Fatigue
   Fear
   Fluid volume deficit
   Fluid volume deficit, high risk for
   Growth and development, altered
   Infection, high risk for
   Injury, high risk for
   Mobility, impaired physical
   Pain
   Pain, chronic
   Skin integrity, impaired
   Skin integrity, impaired, high risk for
   Tissue perfusion, altered (specify type) (renal, cerebral, cardiopulmonary, gastrointestinal, peripheral)
   Sexual dysfunction

3. **Examples of objective data for documentation**

   Vital signs
   Swelling
   Use of oxygen
   Results of blood tests (e.g., HCT, HGB)
   Weight
   Cough, chills
   Shortness of breath
   Jaundiced sclera
   Date of last hospitalization
   Pain, _____ location

4. **Examples of the assessment of the data**

   Acute crisis
   Febrile
   Dehydration
   IV of _____ as ordered; patent and infusing
   Productive cough
   Abdominal (or other) site of pain
   Patient needs analgesia for pain relief
   Enlarged spleen
   Pain

5. **Examples of potential medical problems for this patient**

   Congestive heart failure
   Renal failure
   Respiratory distress/pneumonia
   Osteomyelitis
   Retinopathy
   Priapism
   Splenomegaly
   Involvement of any major organ
   Infections/sepsis
   Delayed growth and sexual maturation
   Complications of blood transfusions
   CVA or cerebral hemorrhage

6. **Examples of the documentation of the potential nursing interventions/actions**

   Comprehensive patient assessment performed
   Pain assessment performed, including site(s), frequency, character
   Emotional support provided to patient, family/caregiver(s)
   Patient/caregiver(s) taught importance of fluid/hydration status
   Assessed site and amount of swelling
   Patient repositioned for comfort
   Care per protocol of stasis ulcers performed; sites without exudate, warmth, or tenderness

Daily weights
Intake and output being monitored
Auscultation of breath sounds completed
Patient repositioned for comfort
Venipunctures obtained as ordered
RN administered ordered analgesic
Vital signs being monitored q hour
ROM exercise completed

7. **Examples of the evaluations of the interventions/actions**

IV patent and site without redness, tenderness, swelling, or other signs of infection/infiltration
Response to new medication positive, without untoward side effects
Temperature rechecked; now _____, within normal range for patient
Pain controlled as verbalized by patient
Caregiver demonstrated correct procedure of use of PCA as taught by RN
Pain relief verbalized after RN administered ordered analgesics
Decreased swelling noted in left knee; had increased ROM at site today
Lab values of _____, within normal range for patient
Abdomen no longer distended
Urinary output within normal range for patient
Patient able to rest between planned interventions
Bowel regimen effective; patient had bowel movement this AM
Patient's intake has improved with offering of more frequent, smaller meals
Weight decreased to _____ from earlier weight of _____ (specify date)
Patient maintaining ordered bed rest
Negative blood cultures
Breath, lung sounds clear on auscultation
Affected joint now without warmth, swelling, or pain
Patient no longer experiencing shortness of breath

Stasis ulcer sites without exudate, warmth, or tenderness

Patient tolerated transfusion of packed red blood cells with no adverse effects

8. **Other services that may be indicated and their associated interventions and goals/outcomes**

Nurse aide

Personal care
ADL assistance
Other duties
Goals:
> Effective personal care provided
> Patient clean and comfortable

Occupational therapy

Evaluation
Conservation-of-energy techniques
Teach safe use of adaptive, assistive devices
ADL retraining
Goals:
> Increased functional mobility
> Uses conservation-of-energy techniques
> Independent ADL

Chaplaincy

Spiritual support offered to patient, family/caregiver(s)
Goals:
> Spiritual support provided to patient, family/caregiver(s)
> Referral to community spiritual resource(s) as indicated

Social work

Assessment of social/emotional factors impacting on health
Financial resource information to patient, family/caregiver(s)
Referral(s) to identified community resources

Goals:
> Problem identification and referral(s) to resources
> Meeting with patient, family prior to discharge to communicate plan
> Referral to community support group

Discharge planning nurse/team

Comprehensive patient evaluation
Communication of identified needs to interdisciplinary team
Referral(s) as indicated based on needs
Goals:
> Evaluation for and referral(s) to identified community resources

9. Nursing goals and outcomes

Daily implementation of care plan, created within
_____ hours of admission and updated and/or
reevaluated q _____ hours or as indicated by patient's condition
Return to self-care or status prior to hospitalization, pain-free with functional mobility and ambulation
Pain, other symptoms controlled
Afebrile, infection controlled
Return to prehospital mobility status
Self-care
Adequate hydration/nutritional status
Patient, family/caregiver(s) able to care for patient
Patient knowledgeable about factors that can precipitate a crisis

10. Potential discharge plans for this patient

Discharge to home; self-care
Discharge to home with caregiver able to care for patient
Discharge to home with community home nursing care follow-up
Discharge to nursing home for continued inpatient skilled care
Symptom-controlled death in hospital

Surgical Care

1. **Assessment of the patient problem**
   Obtain subjective data from the patient, family, or caregiver(s)

2. **Associated nursing diagnoses**
   Activity intolerance
   Activity intolerance, high risk for
   Anxiety
   Breathing pattern, ineffective
   Constipation
   Fatigue
   Fear
   Fluid volume deficit, high risk for
   Infection, high risk for
   Nutrition, altered: less than body requirements
   Oral mucous membrane, altered
   Pain
   Pain, chronic
   Role performance, altered
   Self-care deficit, bathing/hygiene
   Self-care deficit, dressing/grooming
   Skin integrity, impaired
   Skin integrity, impaired, high risk for
   Tissue perfusion, altered (specify type) (renal, cerebral, cardiopulmonary, gastrointestinal, peripheral)
   Urinary elimination, altered patterns

3. **Examples of objective data for documentation**
   Allergies
   Vital signs
   Weight
   Visitor's presence
   Dietary information

Intake and output
Vomiting
Lab or x-ray results
Crying, grimacing
Use of dentures/glasses/contact lenses
Position of patient
Loose or liquid stools
Abdominal distention
Residual urine

4. Examples of the assessment of the data

Unstable vital signs
Acute abdominal (or other) pain
Weight loss
Patent urinary catheter
Pain relief as evidenced by _____
High or low blood pressure
Febrile
Uncontrolled pain/other symptoms
Impaction; unable to evacuate stool
Patient upset, uncomfortable
Visual and/or hearing deficit(s)
Decreased output of _____ this hour (specify time)
Anxiety decreased after questions
answered/explanation given
Physician notified of change identified

5. Examples of potential medical problems for this patient

Anesthesia problems
Pneumonia
Thrombophlebitis
Urinary tract infection
Wound infection
Hemorrhage
Dehiscence
Electrolyte imbalance

6. **Examples of the documentation of potential nursing interventions/actions**

Comprehensive nursing assessment completed per facility protocol

RN conducted preoperative teaching with patient and family/caregiver(s); included importance of postoperative verbal orientation to time, place, person, and their roles in assisting during the hospital stay

Patient with sensory deficits shown physical layout of room

Patient taught importance of deep breathing and coughing postoperatively

Patient taught relaxation exercises and demonstrated to RN

Assessed patient on unit postoperatively

Pain, nausea, other symptom evaluation completed

Mouth care provided to patient for comfort

Incentive spirometry used to facilitate lung expansion

Vital signs obtained per physician order(s)

Patient dangled at bedside with assistance

Enteral feedings being given via pump per physician order(s)/hospital protocol

Evaluated postoperative wound site and wound dressing(s)

Intake and output being monitored q hour

Foley catheter care provided

RN auscultated lungs, encouraged patient to cough, deep breathe

Ordered ice chips being given to patient by family

Administered ordered analgesic and antiemetic

Suppository administered as ordered for complaints of gas pain

Comfort measure of back rub provided to patient

Nasogastric tube care as ordered

Patient's position being changed q 2 hours

Assessed hydration/nutritional status

Daily weights

Emotional support provided to patient and family

Patient observed for signs, symptoms of infections

postoperatively (wound, lungs, urinary, thrombophlebitis)

Physician notified of change in patient's condition (specify)

Abdomen splinted with pillow to facilitate coughing/decrease pain

Antiembolus/elastic hose in place

Lotion applied to dry skin areas of legs and feet

Venipuncture(s) obtained as ordered

Patient oriented to time, place, and person

Hospital chaplain contacted as family requested

Patient reassured of location postoperatively

Postoperative assessment of pain (amount, character, frequency, site[s]), and relief interventions as ordered

Stoma site cleansed and cared for per orders

Suctioning provided per protocol

IV antibiotic of _____ hung as ordered

Patient taught to cough/expectorate effectively

Treatment of chest physical therapy/postural drainage provided

Suppository of ordered antipyretic administered

IV site changed per protocol

Taught patient's family appropriate skills to be able to assist in care

Obtained urine specimen for culture and sensitivity

7. **Examples of the evaluations of the interventions/actions**

Pain relief expressed after administration of ordered analgesic

Lab value of _____, within normal range for patient

Family/caregiver demonstrated correct procedure as taught by RN

Temperature rechecked at _____ PM, after antipyretic; now _____

Patient had first postoperative bowel movement (small, formed)

Patient using PCA pump as taught preoperatively

Pain (or any other symptom) now controlled by

_____

No evidence of impaction on exam; patient has hemorrhoids
Weight decreased since yesterday (specify dates)
Skin integrity remains intact; continue protocol and q 2 hour position changes
Patient able to rest after backrub
Patient is coughing and deep breathing as taught
Patient's weight remains stable on tube feedings
Catheter patent and draining
Unexpected amount of bloody drainage for third postoperative day—reported to physician
Patient ambulating halls with assistance of one
Patient wants food; is tired of clear liquids—physician notified

8. **Other services that may be indicated and their associated interventions and goals/outcomes**

   Nurse aide

   Personal care
   ADL assistance
   Other duties
   Goals:
   > Effective personal care provided
   > Patient clean and comfortable

   Physical therapy

   Evaluation
   Chest physical therapy
   Teach safe use of assistive devices
   Therapeutic and strengthening exercises
   Postsurgery conditioning and endurance training
   Goals:
   > Pulmonary program achieved
   > Safely using assistive devices
   > Return to prior level of mobility; patient able to demonstrate home exercise program taught

Chaplaincy

Spiritual support offered to patient,
family/caregiver(s)
Goals:

Spiritual support provided to patient,
family/caregiver(s)
Referral to community spiritual resource(s) as
indicated

Social work

Assessment of social/emotional factors impacting on
health
Financial resource information to patient,
family/caregiver(s)
Referral(s) to identified community resources
Goals:

Problem identification and referral(s) to resources
Meeting with patient, family prior to discharge to
communicate plan

Discharge planning nurse/team

Comprehensive patient evaluation
Communication of identified needs to team member
Referral(s) to community resources
Goals:

Evaluation for and referral to identified
community resources

9. **Nursing goals and outcomes**

Daily implementation of care plan, created within
_____ hours of admission and updated and/or
reevaluated q _____ hours or as indicated by patient's
condition
Return to self-care or status prior to hospitalization,
pain-free with functional mobility and ambulation
Ambulatory
Self-care
Voiding/bowel movements resumed
Afebrile/without infection(s)
Diet resumed

10. Potential discharge plans for this patient

Nursing home placement for continued care
Discharge to home; self-care
Discharge to home with community home nursing
services follow-up
Symptom-controlled death in hospital

Tracheostomy Care

◆

1. **Assessment of the patient problem**

   Obtain subjective data from the patient, family, or caregiver(s)

2. **Associated nursing diagnoses**

   Airway clearance, ineffective
   Anxiety
   Body image disturbance
   Communication, impaired verbal
   Fear
   Home maintenance management, impaired
   Infection, high risk for
   Knowledge deficit (specify)
   Nutrition, altered: less than body requirements
   Pain
   Skin integrity, impaired
   Swallowing, impaired

3. **Examples of objective data for documentation**

   Vital signs
   Weight
   Visitor's presence
   Bleeding from tracheostomy site
   Method of communication

4. **Examples of the assessment of the data**

   Unstable vital signs
   Anxiety decreased after suctioning
   Weight less than yesterday, or other specified date
   Patient able to communicate effectively with pen and paper
   Patient able to communicate effectively after assessment visit with speech-language pathologist, who left word cards at bedside

5. **Examples of potential medical problems for this patient**

Infection
Aspiration pneumonia
Erosion through artery
Tracheitis
Asphyxia
Respiratory distress

6. **Examples of the documentation of potential nursing interventions/actions**

Stoma site cleansed per protocol (specify)
Emotional support given to patient and family
Patient suctioned
Observed for signs, symptoms of tracheitis
Intake and output being monitored
Amount, type of secretions being monitored
Safety feature of clamp taped to head of bed
Teaching begun with patient/caregiver regarding suctioning technique
Breath sounds evaluated after suctioning to determine effectiveness
Emotional support provided to patient/family
Cuff deflated as ordered per facility protocol
Fluid of patient's choice encouraged
Listened to patient's concerns after patient was notified of pathology report
Comfort measure of back massage provided
Reassured patient of call bell system, should help be needed
Assessed stoma site for bleeding, other drainage, skin condition
Daily weights
Patient/family cautioned to avoid use of aerosol sprays,   powders, and other particles that could be aspirated
Changed ties with assistance of _____
Monitored and reported results of ABGs

Bowel function/comfort being maintained
For patient on tube feeding, placement and residual checked prior to feeding, and head of bed elevated
Contacted hospital chaplain at patient's request
Team meeting held regarding patient's home situation and impending discharge
Amount of bloody drainage reported to physician

7. **Examples of the evaluations of the interventions/actions**

Patient comfortable; pain relieved after administration of analgesic
Patient not experiencing shortness of breath now
Temperature within normal range for patient
Patient's weight is being maintained on tube feeding regimen
Family, patient express comfort level with new discharge plan
Patient and spouse demonstrated proper suctioning techniques as taught by RN
No evidence of impaction
Catheter patent; amber urine draining into drainage bag
Patient now able to rest between planned interventions
Wound site without crust, exudate, or unusual redness
Stoma healing occurring
Dressing showed minimal amount of bright red bleeding

8. **Other services that may be indicated and their associated interventions and goals/outcomes**

Nurse aide
Personal care
ADL assistance
Other duties
Goals:
 Effective personal care provided
 Patient clean and comfortable

Physical therapy
- Evaluation
- Chest physical therapy
- Therapeutic exercise regimen
- ROM
- Bed mobility exercises as tolerated
- Strengthening exercises
- Teach use of assistive devices as indicated

Goals:
- Pulmonary program goals achieved
- Increased mobility
- Patient/family knowledgeable about home exercise regimen
- Patient able to safely use assistive devices

Occupational therapy

Evaluation

Functional mobility

Conservation-of-energy techniques

ADL training

Upper extremity therapeutic exercises and activities

Goals:
- Patient using conservation-of-energy techniques
- Patient able to use ADL assistive devices
- Functional mobility improved or maintained

Speech-language pathology

Comprehensive speech/swallowing evaluation

Development and teaching of communication system

Goals:
- Effective, safe swallowing
- Patient able to communicate
- Functional communication system in place

Chaplaincy

Spiritual support offered to patient, family/caregiver(s)

Goals:
- Spiritual support provided to patient, family/caregiver(s)

Referral to community spiritual resource(s) as indicated

Social work

Assessment of emotional/social factors impacting on health
Financial resource information to patient, family, caregiver(s)
Referral(s) to identified community resources
Goals:

Problem identification and referral(s) to resources
Meeting with patient/family to ensure communication of plan

Discharge planning nurse/team

Comprehensive patient evaluation
Communication of evaluation with other team members, patient, family/caregiver(s)
Referral(s) to community resources
Goals:

Evaluation for and referral(s) to identified community resources

9. **Nursing goals and outcomes**

Daily implementation of care plan, created within _____ hours of admission and updated and/or reevaluated q _____ hours or as indicated by patient's condition
Return to self-care or status prior to hospitalization, pain-free with functional mobility and ambulation
Patent airway
Adequate gas exchange
Patient or caregiver taught and able to demonstrate tracheostomy care
Respiratory status stable
Adequate hydration/nutritional status maintained
Infection-free or infection controlled
Patient without complaint of dyspnea

10. **Potential discharge plans for this patient**

Nursing home placement for continued skilled care and therapy

Discharge to home with patient/family able to assume care

Discharge to home with referral for home nursing and therapy services

Symptom-controlled death in inpatient setting

Urinary Catheter Care

◆

1. **Assessment of the patient problem**
   Obtain subjective data from the patient, family, or caregiver(s)

2. **Associated nursing diagnoses**
   Incontinence, functional
   Incontinence, reflex
   Incontinence, stress
   Incontinence, total
   Incontinence, urge
   Infection, high risk for
   Injury, high risk for
   Mobility, impaired physical
   Pain
   Pain, chronic
   Self-care deficit, bathing/hygiene
   Self-care deficit, toileting
   Trauma, high risk for
   Urinary elimination, altered patterns
   Urinary retention

3. **Examples of objective data for documentation**
   Bladder distention
   Residual urine
   Vital signs
   Presence of indwelling catheter and drainage bag
   Hematuria
   Urinary output, _____ cc
   Positive urinary culture of _____
   Suprapubic area tenderness
   Fever, chills
   Use of assistive devices
   Family/caregiver(s) accompanying patient
   Medications that patient takes at home
   Nocturia
   Urinary frequency

4. **Examples of the assessment of the data**

Patent urinary catheter
Alert, oriented x3
Physician notified of identified changes
Suprapubic catheter care site given per facility
protocol/physician order(s)
Patient with history of UTIs readmitted to unit for IV
antibiotics
Intake and output within normal range for patient

5. **Examples of potential medical problems for this patient**

Urinary tract infection
Cystitis
Urethritis
Bladder spasms

6. **Examples of the documentation of potential nursing interventions/actions**

Temperature rechecked; now _____, within normal
range for patient
Catheter #_____ , _____ cc changed without problem;
150 cc residual noted
Patient expressed increased comfort after first dose of
antispasmodic
Catheter irrigated with 30 cc normal saline solution
(NSS) prn per physician order(s)
Family taught care of catheter prior to discharge
Urine specimen obtained for culture and sensitivity
Fluids of patient's preference being offered every hour

7. **Examples of the evaluations of the interventions/actions**

Negative urinary cultures
Bladder no longer distended
Vital signs within normal range for patient
Urinary output within normal range for patient
Caregiver now demonstrates correct procedure of
_____ as taught by RN

Afebrile
Patient pain-free after administration of ordered
analgesic
Patent urinary catheter draining (description of urine)

8. **Other services that may be indicated and their
   associated interventions and goals/outcomes**

   Nurse aide

   Personal care
   ADL assistance
   Other duties
   Goals:
   > Effective personal care provided
   > Patient clean and comfortable

   Chaplaincy

   > Spiritual support offered to patient,
   > family/caregiver(s)
   Goals:
   > Spiritual support provided to patient,
   > family/caregiver(s)

   Social work

   Assessment of emotional/social factors impacting on
   health
   Financial resource information to patient/family
   Goals:
   > Problem identification and referral(s) to
   > appropriate resources

   Discharge planning nurse/team

   Comprehensive patient evaluation
   Communication of identified needs to team
   Referral(s) to community resources
   Goals:
   > Referral information communicated to RN in
   > facility where patient will be living after discharge
   > Meeting with patient, family prior to discharge to
   > communicate plan and facilitate continuity of care

9. **Nursing goals and outcomes**

   Daily implementation of care plan, created within
   _____ hours of admission and updated and/or
   reevaluated q _____ hours or as indicated by patient's
   condition
   Return to self-care or status prior to hospitalization,
   pain-free with functional mobility and ambulation
   Patent catheter
   Infection-free or infection controlled
   Patient or family member able to care for patient on
   discharge
   Hydration adequate
   Afebrile

10. **Potential discharge plans for this patient**

    Nursing home placement
    Discharge to home with support of community home
    nursing services
    Discharge to home; self-care without indwelling
    urinary catheter

Wound Care

1. Assessment of the patient problem

Obtain subjective data from the patient, family, or caregiver(s)

2. Associated nursing diagnoses

Body image disturbance
Body temperature, altered, high risk for
Constipation
Denial, ineffective
Disuse syndrome, high risk for
Fatigue
Fluid volume deficit (1)
Fluid volume deficit (2)
Fluid volume deficit, high risk for
Infection, high risk for
Mobility, impaired physical
Nutrition, altered: less than body requirements
Pain
Pain, chronic
Powerlessness
Self-care deficit, bathing/hygiene
Self-care deficit, dressing/grooming
Self-care deficit, feeding
Self-care deficit, toileting
Sensory/perceptual alterations (specify) (visual, auditory, kinesthetic, gustatory, tactile, olfactory)
Sexuality patterns, altered
Skin integrity, impaired
Skin integrity, impaired, high risk for
Spiritual distress (distress of the human spirit)
Tissue integrity, impaired
Trauma, high risk for
Urinary elimination, altered patterns

3. **Examples of objective data for documentation**
   Vital signs
   Wound site(s), description, and location
   Tears, crying
   IV solution, rate ordered, site
   Presence of urinary or other catheter(s)
   Breath sounds
   Level of consciousness
   Vomiting
   Blood glucose levels
   Weight
   Visitors/caregivers accompanying patient
   Intake and output
   Skin color

4. **Examples of the assessment of the data**
   Unstable vital signs
   Alert, oriented x3
   Upset, depressed
   IV infusing
   Patent urinary catheter
   Change noted in breath sounds
   Physician notified of change
   Wound healing as evidenced by _____

5. **Examples of potential medical problems for this patient**
   Wound infection
   Cellulitis
   Diabetes mellitus
   Tissue necrosis
   Chronic stasis ulcers
   Peripheral vascular disease
   Amputation
   Dermatitis

6. Examples of the documentation of potential nursing interventions/actions

Initial wound assessment(s) completed on admission

Wound site(s) cultured

Foot soaked in _____ solution as ordered

Site wrapped with _____ as ordered

Patient taught regarding new antibiotic regimen

Patient started on pain control regimen of _____

Teaching of care of wound site begun with patient and caregiver

Safety measures regarding decreased sensation in lower extremity taught to caregiver (e.g., avoid use of heating pads)

Patient administered first dose of new antibiotic for infected ulcer(s), wound(s) of _____

Support hose applied

Dressing changed per protocol of _____

IV solution of _____ started

Removed dressing

Assessed for signs of decreased circulation

Evaluated healing progress

Wound site culture obtained and sent to lab

Assessed hydration/nutritional status

Patient medicated with pain medication prior to dressing change

Pain assessment performed

Taught patient, family/caregiver(s) prescribed wound care and dressing procedure(s)

7. Examples of the evaluations of the interventions/actions

Pain relief expressed after po administration of analgesic

Decreased swelling noted in left lower leg; measurement now _____

Healing, granulation seen in wound site

Color of skin noted to be pink around wound site
Lab value of _____, within normal range for patient
Temperature rechecked at _____ PM; now _____, within normal range
Pain controlled as evidenced by _____
Learning barrier of _____ identified; will teach another family member
Patient not vomiting after administration of antiemetic suppository
Family/caregiver demonstrated correct procedure as taught
Wound site without swelling, redness, or exudate

8. **Other services that may be indicated and their associated interventions and goals/outcomes**

Nurse aide

Personal care
ADL assistance
Other duties
Goals:
    Effective personal care provided
    Patient verbalizes comfort and feeling of well-being
    Assistance with ADL provided

Chaplaincy

Spiritual support offered to patient, family/caregiver(s)
Goals:
    Spiritual support provided to patient, family/caregiver(s)
    Referral to community spiritual resource(s) as indicated

Social work

Assessment of social and emotional factors
Counseling
Financial assistance

Referral(s) to resources as identified by needs
assessment
Goals:
    Resources identified and referral(s) made to
    community programs

Discharge planning nurse/team

Comprehensive evaluation of patient's needs
Home nursing care referral
Goals:
    Patient, family prepared for discharge
    Patient discharged to appropriate level of care
    setting

9. **Nursing goals and outcomes**

    Daily implementation of care plan, created within
    _____ hours of admission and updated and/or
    reevaluated q _____ hours or as indicated by patient's
    condition
    Return to self-care or status prior to hospitalization,
    pain-free with functional mobility and ambulation
    Wound healing
    Wound with decreased swelling
    Wound infection-free
    Patient/family/caregiver taught and able to care for
    patient/self
    Compliance to regimens demonstrated by
    patient/family while a patient

10. **Potential discharge plans for this patient**

    Discharge to home; returned to self-care status
    Nursing home placement for continued care
    Discharge to home with home nursing services for
    continued care

PART THREE

HOSPICE CARE
DOCUMENTATION
GUIDELINES

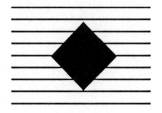

Hospice Care

◆

1. **Assessment of the patient problem**

   Obtain subjective data from the patient, family, or
   caregiver(s)

2. **Associated nursing diagnoses**

   Activity intolerance
   Activity intolerance, high risk for
   Adjustment, impaired
   Airway clearance, ineffective
   Anxiety
   Aspiration, high risk for
   Body image disturbance
   Body temperature, altered, high risk for
   Bowel incontinence
   Breathing pattern, ineffective
   Cardiac output, decreased
   Communication, impaired verbal
   Constipation
   Constipation, colonic
   Disuse syndrome, high risk for
   Diversional activity deficit
   Family processes, altered
   Fatigue
   Fear
   Fluid volume deficit
   Fluid volume excess
   Gas exchange, impaired
   Grieving, anticipatory
   Growth and development, altered
   Incontinence, functional
   Incontinence, total
   Infection, high risk for
   Mobility, impaired physical
   Nutrition, altered: less than body requirements
   Oral mucous membrane, altered

Pain
Pain, chronic
Parenting, altered
Role performance, altered
Self-care deficit, bathing/hygiene
Self-care deficit, dressing/grooming
Self-care deficit, feeding
Self-care deficit, toileting
Self-esteem disturbance
Sensory/perceptual alterations (auditory)
Sexuality patterns, altered
Skin integrity, impaired
Skin integrity, impaired, high risk for
Sleep pattern disturbance
Social interaction, impaired
Social isolation
Spiritual distress (distress of the human spirit)
Swallowing, impaired
Thermoregulation, ineffective
Thought processes, altered
Tissue integrity, impaired
Tissue perfusion, altered (specify type) (renal, cerebral, cardiopulmonary, gastrointestinal, peripheral)
Urinary elimination, altered patterns
Urinary retention

3. **Examples of objective data for documentation**
   Vital signs
   Level of consciousness
   Loose or liquid stools
   Abdominal distention
   Cheyne-Stokes or irregular breathing pattern
   Residual urine
   Impaction
   Presence of urinary catheter
   Diaphoresis
   Family at bedside
   Restlessness
   Dyspnea

Presence of hospice volunteer, chaplain, other team members
Weight
Lower extremity edema
Patient's pet in to visit and at bedside per protocol

4. **Examples of the assessment of the data**

   Unstable vital signs (e.g., BP high or low, febrile, change in vital signs)
   Alert, oriented x3
   Unresponsive
   Impaction; unable to evacuate stool
   Upset, depressed, uncomfortable
   Patent urinary catheter
   Weight change
   Pain relief

5. **Examples of potential medical problems for this patient**

   Urinary tract infection
   Pneumonia or other lung process
   Thrombophlebitis
   Pulmonary embolism
   Trauma (falls)
   Skin breakdown
   Obstruction
   Oncology complications
   Other complications based on original pathology

6. **Examples of the documentation of potential nursing interventions/actions**

   Presented hospice philosophy
   Assessed wishes and expectations of patient, family/caregiver(s) regarding care
   Assessed family or caregiver(s) for availability of support and care
   Psychosocial assessment of patient and family performed regarding disease and prognosis

Taught family or caregiver(s) care of patient

Assessed bowel habits and regimen; implemented program as needed

Assessed pain and other symptoms, including site(s), duration, characteristics, relief measures

Taught care of the bedridden

Completed assessment of cardiovascular, pulmonary, and respiratory status

Implemented pain, other symptom control measures

Assessed and monitored hydration/nutritional status

Implemented and taught new pain and other symptom control medication regimen and other comfort measures

Assisted patient with guided imagery or progressive muscle relaxation exercises to assist in control of anxiety or pain relief

Taught family regarding safe transfer of patient from chair to bed

Family and other caregivers attended team conference regarding patient's request to return home; plans made to achieve that goal

Comfort measures being provided (e.g., massages, music of choice, favorite meals that family members bring in and that patient can tolerate)

Patient's daily regimen being maintained as much as possible (could include makeup applications, personalized hair care, and manicures/pedicures)

Family is providing patient's own bed linens and clothing from home

Diet counseling completed for patient with anorexia

Checked for and removed impaction(s) as needed

Assessed patency of condom catheter or indwelling catheter

Taught caregiver(s) symptom and pain control measures

Measured abdominal girth for ascites and edema; documented sites and amount

Oxygen on at _____ liters per nasal cannula

Assessed mental status, sleep disturbance changes

Taught catheter care to caregiver(s)

Ongoing assessment of skin integrity

7. **Examples of the evaluations of the interventions/actions**

No evidence of impaction
Patient able to sleep through night after administration of pain medication and comfort measures
Urinary output within normal limits for patient
Skin remains clear, dry, pink; no evidence of breakdown of skin integrity
Abdomen no longer distended; bowel sounds within normal limits for patient
Patient no longer vomiting after administration of antiemetic suppository

8. **Other services that may be indicated and their associated interventions and goals/outcomes**

Volunteer support

Core service unique to hospice care; indicated based on patient and family, nursing and volunteer coordinator assessment of patient and family
Responsibilities vary; may include personal care, companionship, running errands, and other needs identified by patient and family

Nurse aide

Personal care
ADL assistance
Other duties
Goals:
    Effective personal care provided
    ADL assistance provided
    Patient clean and comfortable

Physical therapy

Evaluation
Teach patient, family, and volunteers safe transfer techniques
Other exercises as based on assessment
Goals:
    Maintenance of function
    Prevention of complications

Occupational therapy

Evaluation
Conservation-of-energy techniques
Assistive device evaluation
Goals:
> Quality of life improved through conservation-of-energy techniques and use of adaptive devices

Speech-language pathology

Speech and swallowing comprehensive evaluation
Alaryngeal speech
Aphasia treatment
Goals:
> Patient able to communicate
> Patient able to swallow

Chaplaincy

Spiritual support offered to patient, family/caregiver(s)
Goals:
> Spiritual support provided to patient, family/caregiver(s)

Social work

Evaluation
Supportive counseling to patient, family/caregiver(s)
Financial assessment and resource identification
Goals:
> Psychosocial support
> Community resources identified

Discharge planning nurse

Comprehensive patient evaluation
Communication of evaluation with other hospice team members, patient, family/caregiver(s)
Referral(s) to community resources
Goals:
> If patient wants to return to home setting, referral made to community hospice program with continuation of plan of care and volunteer support

9. **Nursing goals and outcomes**
   Daily implementation of care plan, created within
   _____ hours of admission and updated and/or
   reevaluated q _____ hours or as indicated by patient's
   condition
   Return to self-care or status prior to hospitalization,
   with functional mobility and ambulation where
   possible
   Support provided to patient and family through death
   Pain and other symptom(s) controlled
   Death with dignity, with loved ones present where
   possible
   Patient comfort through death

10. **Potential discharge plans for this patient**
    Referral to home hospice program
    Death in facility with pain and other symptoms
    controlled; loved ones present at death with
    bereavement counseling begun
    Death in home setting

PART FOUR

MATERNAL/CHILD CARE DOCUMENTATION GUIDELINES

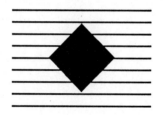

Acquired Immune Deficiency Syndrome (AIDS) (Care of the Child with)

◆

1. **Assessment of the patient problem**

   Obtain subjective data from the patient, parents, or caregiver(s)

2. **Associated nursing diagnoses**

   Adjustment, impaired

   Airway clearance, ineffective

   Anxiety

   Body image disturbance

   Body temperature, altered, high risk for

   Bowel incontinence

   Cardiac output, decreased

   Coping, ineffective family: compromised

   Coping, ineffective family: disabling

   Coping, ineffective individual

   Fatigue

   Fear

   Fluid volume deficit

   Fluid volume deficit, high risk for

   Gas exchange, impaired

   Grieving, anticipatory

   Growth and development, altered

   Injury, high risk for

   Infection, high risk for

   Knowledge deficit (self-care)

   Nutrition, altered: less than body requirements

   Oral mucous membrane, altered

   Pain

   Pain, chronic

   Powerlessness

   Protection, altered

   Role performance, altered

   Self-care deficit, bathing/hygiene

   Self-care deficit, dressing/grooming

Self-care deficit, feeding
Self-care deficit, toileting
Sensory/perceptual alterations (specify) (visual,
auditory, kinesthetic, gustatory, tactile, olfactory)
Sexual dysfunction
Sexuality patterns, altered
Skin integrity, impaired
Skin integrity, impaired, high risk for
Social isolation
Spiritual distress (distress of the human spirit)
Swallowing, impaired
Thought processes, altered
Tissue integrity, impaired, high risk for
Tissue perfusion, altered (specify type) (renal, cerebral,
cardiopulmonary, gastrointestinal, peripheral)
Urinary elimination, altered patterns

3. **Examples of objective data for documentation**
Pain
Height, weight
Date of last hospitalization
General appearance
Vital signs
Level of consciousness
Diarrhea
Tears, crying
Results of bone marrow aspiration, other diagnostic
tests
Wheezing, stridor, grunting, nasal flaring, retractions,
head bobbing, seesaw breathing
IV solution, rate infusing, site description
Blood values
Immunizations (to date)
Dyspnea, SOB
Occult blood
Thin; weight plotted on growth chart
Lung, breath sounds
Lymph nodes (enlarged)
Sputum production, frequency, amount, color,

character
Use of oxygen
Presence of parents, other visitors
Absence of parents, other visitors
Frequency of illness
Skin eruptions (e.g., rash, acne)
Diaper rash and description
White areas in mouth
Thrush
Is child at proper milestone for growth and
development for age?

4. **Examples of the assessment of the data**
   Unstable vital signs (e.g., low BP, febrile)
   Alert, oriented x3
   Upset
   IV infusing
   Failure to thrive
   Pain, controlled or uncontrolled
   Unable to eat; thrush in mouth
   Joint limitations
   Weight loss or gain
   Small for gestational age
   Changes in lung sounds
   Patent catheter
   Repeated infections
   Recurrent ear infections
   Productive cough

5. **Examples of potential medical problems for this patient**
   Urinary tract infection
   Kaposi's sarcoma
   Pneumocystis carinii pneumonia
   Endocarditis
   Encephalitis
   Meningitis
   Myocarditis
   Candidal infections

Tuberculosis
Otitis media
Anemias
Lymphomas
Herpes
Cytomegalovirus
Chorioretinitis
Salmonella
Hepatitis
Cardiomyopathy
Leukemia
Squamous cell carcinomas of rectum or mouth
Miscellaneous other protozoal, fungal, viral, or bacterial infections
Sepsis
Allergic reactions to therapies
Other cancers

6. **Examples of the documentation of potential nursing interventions/actions**

Taught parents/caregiver(s) care of child
RN began teaching muscle relaxation techniques to child
Parents taught how to evaluate pain using visual pain scales
Observed for signs of oral thrush (candidiasis)
Emotional support provided to child and family
Strict "universal precautions" being maintained for all body fluids
Nutritional education provided for parents (i.e., foods high in calories and nutrition)

7. **Examples of the evaluations of the interventions/actions**

Temperature rechecked at _____ PM; now _____
Successful plan as shown by _____
Patient verbalizes comfort after administration of ordered analgesia and repositioning
Gamma globulin injection administered as ordered

with no untoward side effect noted
No vomiting; able to take sips of juices of choice

8. **Other services that may be indicated and their associated interventions and goals/outcomes**

Nurse aide

Personal care
ADL assistance
Other duties
Goals:
> Effective personal hygiene
> ADL assistance provided
> Patient clean and comfortable
> Respite care for parents

Physical therapy

Evaluation
Strengthening exercises
Passive/active exercises
Transfer techniques
Chest percussion and postural drainage
Goals:
> Increased function and mobility
> Family able to perform exercises taught before discharge
> Prevention of complications

Occupational therapy

Evaluation
Conservation-of-energy techniques
Adaptive or assistive devices as indicated for child's needs
ADL training program
Teach alternative skills, diversional activities
Goals:
> Patient using conservation-of-energy techniques taught
> Quality of life improved through techniques used
> Family/child able to use techniques taught before discharge

Chaplaincy

Spiritual support offered to patient,
family/caregiver(s)
Goals:
    Spiritual support provided to patient,
    family/caregiver(s)
    Referral to community spiritual resource(s) as
    indicated

Social work

Assessment of emotional and social factors impacting
on health
Counseling
Financial assistance
Alternative placement as needed
Food assistance program referral
Goals:
    Problems, resources identified

Discharge planning nurse

Community resource evaluation based on child's
needs
Referral to support group for parents/child
Hospice referral where appropriate
Goals:
    Home nursing care or hospice referral completed
    prior to discharge

9. **Nursing goals and outcomes**

    Daily implementation of care plan, created within
        _____ hours of admission and updated and/or
    reevaluated q _____ hours or as indicated by patient's
    condition
    Symptom and infection control; patient pain-free, or
    pain controlled; other symptoms controlled
    Functional independence for as long as possible;
    comfort and curative (to specific infection/problem)
    and palliative measures

10. Potential discharge plans for this patient

Discharge to home

Follow-up at home with home health services for nursing care and/or continued therapy program

Patient death in inpatient facility with dignity, comfort, support by friends and family, and with symptoms controlled through death

Referral of family/significant other(s) to hospice program for continued palliative care directed toward effective symptom management

Antepartal Care

1. **Assessment of the patient problem**

   Obtain subjective data from the patient, family, or caregiver(s)

2. **Associated nursing diagnoses**

   Activity intolerance
   Activity intolerance, high risk for
   Anxiety
   Body image disturbance
   Cardiac output, decreased
   Constipation
   Diversional activity deficit
   Fatigue
   Family processes, altered
   Fear
   Grieving, anticipatory
   Grieving, dysfunctional
   Growth and development, altered
   Infection, high risk for
   Injury, high risk for
   Knowledge deficit (related to process causing admission)
   Nutrition, altered: high risk for more than body requirements
   Nutrition, altered: less than body requirements
   Nutrition, altered: more than body requirements
   Pain
   Parental role conflict
   Parenting, altered
   Parenting, altered, high risk for
   Role performance, altered
   Sexual dysfunction
   Sexuality patterns, altered
   Skin integrity, impaired

Skin integrity, impaired, high risk for
Sleep pattern disturbance
Spiritual distress (distress of the human spirit)

3. **Examples of objective data for documentation**
   Vital signs
   Level of consciousness
   Tears, crying
   Urinalysis results
   Weights
   Site(s) of edema
   Intake and output
   Lab, ultrasound, other diagnostic results
   IV solution, rate, site location and description
   Bleeding
   Contractions
   Activity level
   Fetal heart rate
   Cough
   Hyperalimenation
   Dyspnea
   Hemoglobin, hematocrit results
   Presence of rales
   Use of continuous electronic fetal monitoring system
   Fundal height
   Fetal presentation (later in pregnancy)
   Leakage of amniotic fluid
   Dilatation

4. **Examples of the assessment of the data**
   Change in vital signs of _____ to _____
   Urinary catheter patent and draining
   Weight loss or gain
   Dyspnea
   Fatigue
   Alert, oriented x3
   Upset, depressed

5. **Examples of potential medical problems for this patient**

   Thrombophlebitis
   CHF
   Diabetes mellitus
   Peripartum cardiomyopathy
   Multiple gestation
   Premature gestation
   Premature labor and delivery
   Spontaneous abortion
   Hypertension
   Hyperemesis
   Pregnancy-induced hypertension
   Ectopic pregnancy
   Cervical incompetence
   Bleeding
   Preeclampsia
   Eclampsia
   Sickle cell anemia
   Infection
   Urinary tract infection
   Placenta previa
   Anemia
   Premature rupture of membranes
   Other

6. **Examples of the documentation of potential nursing interventions/actions**

   Patient repositioned into semi-Fowler's position
   Patient care planned with frequent rest periods
   Elastic stockings applied
   RN noted maternal contractions now being monitored
   RN taught patient about conservation-of-energy techniques
   Daily weights
   Comfort measure of backrub provided
   ROM exercises performed on patient on strict bed rest and prolonged hospitalization

RN obtained ECG strip and alerted physician of change

Medications administered as ordered (specify)

Emotional support provided to patient and caregiver

Diet of _____ taught to patient and caregiver

Oxygen administered for dyspnea at _____ liters per order

Explanation of procedure _____ given to patient

Venipuncture(s) obtained as ordered

Comprehensive nursing assessment completed on admission

RN obtained fetal monitoring strip and alerted physician of change

Patient assessed for changes in blood pressure readings

7. **Examples of the evaluations of the interventions/actions**

Changes in blood pressure identified; physician notified

Patient diuresing

Patient shows weight loss/gain of _____, since (specify date)

Blood pressure decreased to _____, within normal range for patient

ECG read by physician; within normal limits for patient

Patient experiencing no shortness of breath

Caregiver able to demonstrate current procedure of _____ as taught by RN

Lab value of _____, within normal range for patient

Patient able to rest between planned interventions

Patient able to sleep after backrub

Family demonstrating understanding of diet program; brought in low-salt favorite foods

Fetal monitor strip reviewed by physician; patient transferred to Labor and Delivery

8. **Other services that may be indicated and their associated interventions and goals/outcomes**

    Nurse aide

    Personal care
    ADL assistance
    Other duties
    Goals:
    >   Effective personal care provided
    >   Patient clean and comfortable

    Chaplaincy

    Spiritual support offered to patient,
    family/caregiver(s)
    Goals:
    >   Spiritual support provided to patient,
    >   family/caregiver(s)
    >   Bereavement support team contacted where
    >   appropriate (loss)

    Social work

    Assessment of emotional/social factors impacting on
    health
    Financial resource information to patient,
    family/caregiver(s)
    Referral(s) to identified community resources (e.g.,
    WIC Program)
    Goals:
    >   Problem identification and referral(s) to
    >   appropriate community resources
    Discharge planning nurse/team
    Comprehensive patient evaluation
    Communication through evaluation and planning
    with other team members, patient, family/caregiver(s)
    Referral(s) to community resources
    Goals:
    >   Patient and family ready for discharge

9. **Nursing goals and outcomes**

    Daily implementation of care plan, created within
    _____ hours of admission and updated and/or
    reevaluated q _____ hours or as indicated by patient's
    condition
    Return to self-care or status prior to hospitalization,
    pain-free with functional mobility and ambulation
    Patient delivers a healthy infant
    Patient is able to verbalize/demonstrate care for her
    infant on discharge
    Patient has a stable cardiorespiratory status
    Patient has an adequate hydration/nutritional status

10. **Potential discharge plans for this patient**

    Discharge to home, still antepartal, with home nursing
    service follow-up
    Discharge postpartum; self-care and able to care for
    infant

Asthma (Care of the Child with)

◆

1. **Assessment of the patient problem**
   Obtain subjective data from the patient, parents, or
   caregiver(s)

2. **Associated nursing diagnoses**
   Activity intolerance
   Activity intolerance, high risk for
   Anxiety
   Breathing pattern, ineffective
   Communication, impaired verbal
   Coping, family: potential for growth
   Family processes, altered
   Fatigue
   Fear
   Fluid volume deficit, high risk for
   Gas exchange, impaired
   Growth and development, altered
   Infection, high risk for
   Knowledge deficit (diagnosis or treatment)
   Sleep pattern disturbance
   Suffocation, high risk for

3. **Examples of objective data for documentation**
   Vital signs (e.g., respiratory rate)
   Grunting
   Audible wheezing
   Fever
   Specific gravity, urine
   Anxious facial expression
   Seesaw respirations
   Head bobbing
   Diaphoresis
   Use of accessory muscles (retractions)
   Flaring nostrils
   Cough (productive or nonproductive)

Presence of family, other caregivers
Absence of family, other caregivers
Presence or absence of wheezing on auscultation
(NOTE: The absence of wheezing can indicate a
worsening condition)
X-ray or other diagnostic tests
Stridor
Cyanosis, circumoral cyanosis

4. **Examples of the assessment of the data**
   Tachycardia
   Febrile
   Productive cough
   IV started and infusing
   Positive sputum culture
   Responsive or nonresponsive to therapy

5. **Examples of potential medical problems for this patient**
   Asphyxia (death)
   Pneumonia
   Respiratory distress
   Atelectasis
   Status asthmaticus bronchiolitis
   Other

6. **Examples of the documentation of potential nursing interventions/actions**
   Comprehensive baseline assessment obtained
   Administered nebulizer treatment with _____ as ordered
   IV started; initial dose of _____ began infusing at _____AM/PM
   Urine collection bag applied to obtain specific gravity
   Temperature was 102.2° F rectally; administered rectal antipyretic as ordered
   Emotional support provided to patient and family
   Juices of choice given to patient at room temperature

Teaching reinforced regarding importance of sound nutrition, adequate hydration, and avoiding known precipitating factors

Patient being reassessed q _____ for respirations, color, wheezing, and other indicators of status of condition

Parent at bedside encouraging patient to cough effectively as taught by RN

Infant placed in position of comfort to improve ventilation (e.g., infant seat, swing)

7. **Examples of the evaluations of the interventions/actions**

   Respiratory rate _____ and character now within normal range for patient

   Patient able to rest on parent's lap between planned interventions

   Patient no longer using accessory muscles and able to nap

   Parent correctly identified medications and their indications for use at home

8. **Other services that may be indicated and their associated interventions and goals/outcomes**

   Nurse aide
   Personal care
   ADL assistance
   Other duties
   Goals:
   > Effective personal care provided
   > Patient clean and comfortable
   > Respite provided for parents/caregiver(s)

   Physical therapy
   Evaluation
   Chest physical therapy
   Postural drainage
   Breathing exercises

Goals:
>Pulmonary program goals achieved
>Patient and family using exercises taught

Occupational therapy

Evaluation
Teach conservation-of-energy techniques
Teach diversional activities
Encourage normal growth and development
Teach caregiver(s) normal milestones to achieve
Goals:
>Patient/parents pacing activities and using
>conservation-of-energy techniques taught
>Patient/parents providing diversional activities in
>accordance with normal growth and development

Chaplaincy
Spiritual support offered to patient,
parents/caregiver(s)
Goals:
>Spiritual support provided to patient,
>parents/caregiver(s)

Social work

Assessment of emotional/social factors impacting on
health
Financial resource information to patient, parents
Referral(s) to community programs
Goals:
>Problem identification; patient and family referred
>to appropriate resources in community

Discharge planning nurse/team
Patient/family evaluation
Communication of findings to other team members
Referral(s) to community health resources
NOTE: If patient and family are referred to a health
program, such as a home nursing agency for home
evaluation, a nursing report is given to the agency to
ensure continuity of care.

Goals:
> Meeting with patient/parents prior to discharge about impending discharge plans and preparation of home with necessary equipment/supplies

9. Nursing goals and outcomes

Daily implementation of care plan, created within _____ hours of admission and updated and/or reevaluated q _____ hours or as indicated by patient's condition

Return to self-care or status prior to hospitalization, pain-free with functional mobility and ambulation

Stable respiratory and other systems status

Infection-free

Family verbalizes care of child with asthma correctly

Family verbalizes purpose of medications, as well as frequency and method of administration

Family verbalizes signs, symptoms of respiratory distress

Parents able to provide needed care at home

Adequate hydration/nutritional status

10. Potential discharge plans for this patient

Discharge to home with parents/caregiver(s) able to care for child

Discharge to home with community nursing follow-up

Cancer (Care of the Child with)

◆

1. **Assessment of the patient problem**

   Obtain subjective data from the patient, parents, or caregiver(s)

2. **Associated nursing diagnoses**

   Activity intolerance
   Activity intolerance, high risk for
   Adjustment, impaired
   Airway clearance, ineffective
   Anxiety
   Aspiration, high risk for
   Body image disturbance
   Body temperature, altered, high risk for
   Breathing pattern, ineffective
   Cardiac output, decreased
   Constipation
   Coping, family: potential for growth
   Coping, ineffective family: compromised
   Denial, ineffective
   Family processes, altered
   Fatigue
   Fear
   Grieving, anticipatory
   Growth and development, altered
   Infection, high risk for
   Injury, high risk for
   Knowledge deficit (diagnosis and treatment)
   Mobility, impaired physical
   Nutrition, altered: less than body requirements
   Oral mucous membrane, altered
   Pain
   Pain, chronic
   Powerlessness
   Parental role conflict
   Parenting, altered

Parenting, altered, high risk for
Role performance, altered
Self-care deficit, bathing/hygiene
Self-care deficit, dressing/grooming
Self-care deficit, feeding
Self-care deficit, toileting
Sensory/perceptual alterations (specify) (visual,
auditory, kinesthetic, gustatory, tactile, olfactory)
Sexuality patterns, altered
Skin integrity, impaired
Skin integrity, impaired, high risk for
Sleep pattern disturbance
Social interaction, impaired
Spiritual distress (distress of the human spirit)
Tissue perfusion, altered (specify type) (renal, cerebral,
cardiopulmonary, gastrointestinal, peripheral)

3. **Examples of objective data for documentation**
   Abdominal girth
   Alopecia
   Vital signs
   Use of accessory muscles to breathe
   Pallor
   Fatigue
   Cough
   Presence of parents/caregiver(s)
   Absence of parents/caregiver(s)
   Vomiting, nausea
   Weight loss
   Crying, tears
   Lab or other diagnostic tests
   Body temperature (fever, below normal)
   Night sweats
   Insomnia
   Diarrhea or constipation
   Blood in stools

4. **Examples of the assessment of the data**
   Unstable vital signs (e.g., BP high or low, febrile,

change in vital signs)
Patent catheter
Weight loss or gain
Pain
Mucosal ulcerations of mouth
Parent and/or patient very tearful

5. **Examples of potential medical problems for this patient**
Drug toxicity
Infertility
Delayed sexual maturation
Metastases
Radiation enteritis or myelitis
Infections
Intestinal obstruction
Neuropathy
Other

6. **Examples of the documentation of potential nursing interventions/actions**
Comprehensive baseline patient assessment completed on admission
Patient offered foods of choice for meals and snacks
Total parenteral nutrition (TPN) explained to parents by RN, pharmacist, and dietitian at conference
RN explained reason for test to patient, parents
Support to patient and family provided by RN
RN administered analgesic as prescribed
Parent taught care regimens; wants to do as much as possible
RN noted oral ulcerations during AM care; reported to physician
Importance of handwashing taught to children visiting patient after school
Intake and output being monitored
Assessment of skin integrity performed; continue q 2 hour position changes to ensure continued skin integrity

RN assisted with intrathecal administration of
_____ at _____ PM

Daily weights

Explanation of ordered therapy given to child and parents

Physician notified of change in patient's status

Child allowed choice between two possible venipuncture sites; blood obtained for ordered tests and sent to lab

Relaxation and guided imagery practiced with child and parents

RN administered ordered antipyretic

IV patent and infusing at ordered rate of _____

RN listened to parents' grief and concerns after pathology report and prognosis discussed by physician

Team meeting held to plan for discharge back to home

RN contacted hospital chaplain at parent's request

Patient evaluated for signs, symptoms of infection

Patient/parents using PCA pump as taught

RN taught skills of _____ to parents for continuation at home

RN assisted with bone marrow aspiration

7. **Examples of the evaluations of the interventions/actions**

Negative (or positive) cultures

Parent demonstrated skills correctly as taught by RN

Pain relief as evidenced by patient not crying; patient smiling and eating

Patient's temperature within normal range after administration of antipyretic

Patient able to rest between planned intervention schedules

Patient no longer using accessory muscles and able to sleep

Patient without signs, symptoms of infection

Patient able to sleep last night; family had brought in

crib animals, favorite sheets, blanket, and pillow from home

Physician notified of weight loss of _____ since (specify date)

Abdomen no longer distended as evidenced by decreasing abdominal girth

Patient able to rest after backrub

IV antibiotic hung and infused without any reaction noted

8. **Other services that may be indicated and their associated interventions and goals/outcomes**

   Nurse aide

   Personal care
   ADL assistance
   Other duties
   Goals:
   > Effective personal care provided
   > Patient clean and comfortable
   > Respite care provided

   Chaplaincy

   Spiritual support offered to child, parents, siblings
   Goals:
   > Spiritual support provided to child, parents, siblings
   > Referral to community spiritual resource(s) as indicated

   Social work

   Assessment of factors impacting on health needs
   Financial resource and other needed information (e.g., American Cancer Society, Ronald McDonald House)
   Referral(s) to identified community resources
   Goals:
   > Problem identification and referral(s) to resources
   > Communication with patient, parents regarding plan prior to discharge

Discharge planning nurse/team

Comprehensive patient evaluation

Referral(s) to community health programs where indicated

Goals:

>   Home nursing care referral accomplished; nurse spoke with nurse at home care program to give report and ensure continuity of care
>
>   Hospice or home care referral per physician order(s)

9. **Nursing goals and outcomes**

Daily implementation of care plan, created within _____ hours of admission and updated and/or reevaluated q _____ hours or as indicated by patient's condition

Return to self-care or status prior to hospitalization, with functional mobility and ambulation where possible

Pain and other symptoms controlled

Child will remain as functionally independent as possible

Child and parents will have effective emotional support that contributes to the therapeutic process

Physiological functions maintained throughout length of illness

Child continues to play and socialize with other children

Child and parents are active participants in care and have input into decisions and choices

Child infection-free or infection is controlled where possible

10. **Potential discharge plans for this patient**

Discharge to home

Discharge to home with home nursing service follow-up

Discharge to home with hospice support through death

Symptom-controlled death with dignity, with family present in hospital

Cystic Fibrosis (Care of the Child with)

◆

1. **Assessment of the patient problem**

   Obtain subjective data from the patient, parents, or caregiver(s)

2. **Associated nursing diagnoses**

   Activity intolerance
   Activity intolerance, high risk for
   Adjustment, impaired
   Airway clearance, ineffective
   Body image disturbance
   Breathing pattern, ineffective
   Cardiac output, decreased
   Constipation
   Coping, family: potential for growth
   Denial, ineffective
   Family processes, altered
   Fatigue
   Fear
   Fluid volume deficit, high risk for
   Gas exchange, impaired
   Grieving, anticipatory
   Growth and development, altered
   Infection, high risk for
   Knowledge deficit (disease and treatment)
   Nutrition altered: less than body requirements
   Pain
   Sexuality patterns, altered
   Social interaction, impaired
   Spiritual distress (distress of the human spirit)
   Suffocation, high risk for

3. **Examples of objective data for documentation**

   Presence of parents, other visitors
   Absence of parents, other visitors
   Vital signs
   Date of last hospitalization

Weight, height
Caloric intake
Amount, character of sputum
Breath sounds
IV solution, rate, site location and description
Results of lab chemistry tests, x-rays, ABGs, other
diagnostic studies
Cyanosis
Vomiting
Wheezing
Shortness of breath
Cough
Clubbing of fingernails
Bowel sounds, hypoactive/hyperactive

4. **Examples of the assessment of the data**
Weight loss of _____ lb
Dyspnea
Fatigue
IV infusing at _____
Changes in breath sounds
Absence of breath sounds

5. **Examples of potential medical problems for this patient**
Prolapse of rectum
Meconium ileus
Ileus
Diabetes mellitus
Cor pulmonale
Hemoptysis
Pneumothorax
GI obstruction
Delayed sexual maturation
Pneumonia
Sinusitis
Respiratory distress
COPD
Inability to digest certain foods
Other

6. **Examples of the documentation of potential nursing interventions/actions**

   Pulmonary therapy of postural drainage with positioning, vibration, and clapping performed by RN

   Parent assisted RN with administration of aerosol therapy treatment

   Emotional support provided to patient and family

   Physician notified of increase in patient's temperature from _____ to _____

   Parent taught regarding importance of high-protein, high-carbohydrate diet

   RN administered enzyme replacements to patient

   Daily weights

7. **Examples of the evaluations of the interventions/actions**

   Patient expectorated large amount of sputum after pulmonary toilet treatments

   Weight of _____ today; increase of _____ lb noted since _____

   Patient able to rest between planned (therapy) interventions

   Parent verbalized relief after patient had a positive response to antibiotic therapy

   Patient able to give aerosol treatment to self

   Parent demonstrates current procedure as taught by RN

   Patient practicing exercises and conservation-of-energy techniques taught

   Patient tolerated all lunch ordered

8. **Other services that may be indicated and their associated interventions and goals/outcomes**

   Nurse aide

   Personal care

   ADL assistance

   Goals:

       Effective personal care provided

       Patient clean and comfortable

Respiratory therapy

Evaluation of learning needs of patient, family
regarding instruction on performing chest physical
therapy, postural drainage, breathing exercises;
administration of treatments
Goals:

Pulmonary status stable and program goals
achieved

Chaplaincy

Spiritual support offered to patient,
parents/caregiver(s)
Goals:

Spriitual support provided to patient,
parents/caregiver(s)

Social work

Assessment of identified problem
Counseling
Financial assistance
Goals:

Resources identified and referral(s) made to
community resources

Discharge planning nurse/team

Evaluation of patient and family needs
Goals:

Parents and child ready for discharge
Community referral(s) initiated (e.g., home nursing
service follow-up)

9. Nursing goals and outcomes

Daily implementation of care plan, created within
_____ hours of admission and updated and/or
reevaluated q _____ hours or as indicated by patient's
condition
Return to self-care or status prior to hospitalization,
pain-free with functional mobility and ambulation
Stable nutritional status
Adequate hydration

Stable respiratory status
Patient/family able to provide pulmonary treatments
Exercise regimen taught, and patient able to comply
Patient compliance with enzyme replacement therapy

10. Potential discharge plans for this patient

Discharge to home; goals achieved; family able to care for child

Diabetes Mellitus (Care of the Child with)

◆

1. **Assessment of the patient problem**

   Obtain subjective data from the patient, parents, or caregiver(s)

2. **Associated nursing diagnoses**

   Adjustment, impaired
   Anxiety
   Body image disturbance
   Denial, ineffective
   Family processes, altered
   Fatigue
   Fear
   Fluid volume deficit, high risk for
   Gas exchange, impaired
   Grieving, anticipatory
   Growth and development, altered
   Infection, high risk for
   Injury, high risk for
   Knowledge deficit (care of child with diabetes mellitus)
   Noncompliance (care regimens)
   Pain
   Sexual dysfunction
   Sexuality patterns, altered
   Skin integrity, impaired, high risk for
   Social interaction, impaired
   Spiritual distress (distress of the human spirit)
   Thought processes, altered

3. **Examples of objective data for documentation**

   Level of consciousness
   Vital signs
   Increased depth, rate of respiration
   Age at initial diagnosis
   Date of most recent hospitalization

Results of glucose tolerance tests
Amount, frequency, type(s) of insulin child takes at home
Time of last insulin injection
Blood glucose levels
Vomiting
IV solution, rate, site location and description
Intake and output
Use of pump; type
Specific gravity
Presence of subcutaneous insulin delivery system
Presence of parents, siblings, others
Absence of parents, others
Sweating
Shallow respirations
Fruity breath
Weight
Dry skin
Presence and level of ketones
Potassium, other electrolyte levels
Tears, crying
Presence or use of continuous infusion pump
Polydipsia
Polyphagia
Polyuria
Weight loss
Dizziness
Blurred vision
Shakiness/tremors

4. **Examples of the assessment of the data**

   Febrile, with temperature of _____
   Change in vital signs
   IV infusing
   Hyperglycemia _____ mg/dl
   Hypoglycemia _____ mg/dl
   Weight loss
   Diuresis

Diabetic ketoacidosis
Education in all aspects of care need reinforcement,
including:
    Signs, symptoms of hypoglycemia/hyperglycemia
    Insulin administration
    Signs, symptoms of infection
    Sick day rules
    Foot care
    Exercise
    Self–home blood glucose monitoring
Excessive thirst, urination
Dehydration
Hypothermia
Hyperventilation

5. **Examples of potential medical problems for this patient**

Hypoxia
Shock
Cerebral edema
Coma
Hypoglycemia
Electrolyte imbalances
Retinopathy
Diabetic ketoacidosis
Acidosis
Renal failure
Thrombosis
Sepsis
Neuropathy
Acute myocardial infarction
Local tissue atrophy
Monilia or other infections
Cardiac arrest
Poor wound healing
Cardiac enlargement
Cardiac hypertrophy
Other

6. **Examples of the documentation of potential nursing interventions/actions**

Assessed for baseline knowledge regarding aspects of care

Emotional support provided to child and parents after test results

RN initiated teaching of facility protocols regarding juvenile diabetes mellitus (type I)

RN taught actions of new insulin ordered

Parent demonstrated skills of insulin preparation and subcutaneous administration as taught by RN

Administered _____ units of _____ insulin sc in site _____

Parents/caregiver/child instructed about use of _____ (blood glucose monitor) with successful return demonstration

Parents/other caregiver/child instructed regarding sick day rules and verbalized sick day rules correctly

Teaching initiated with parents and child regarding aspects of diet

Venipuncture obtained for ordered tests

Intake and output being monitored

IV site care provided per facility protocol

Urine checked for ketones, prior to breakfast or with BS over 240 mg/dl

Cardiac monitoring continuing because of potassium results obtained

7. **Examples of the evaluations of the interventions/actions**

IV of _____ patent and infusing at ordered rate of _____

Blood glucose of _____, within normal range for patient

Parent demonstrated correct procedure of _____ as taught

Weight has increased to _____ lb since admission

Teaching on mixing insulins progressing; drawn up as demonstrated by RN; patient will attempt self-

injection this PM
Child able to test urine as taught

8. **Other services that may be indicated and their associated interventions and goals/outcomes**

Diabetes nurse educator

Assessment of baseline knowledge of child and family
Teaching on all aspects of care related to diabetes
mellitus
Goals:

Child ultimately able to care for self
Family/caregiver(s) knowledgeable in survival
skills
Referral(s) to community support resources
Referred to local support groups of the Juvenile
Diabetes Association

Nurse aide

Personal care
ADL assistance
Other duties
Goals:

Effective personal hygiene
Patient clean and comfortable

Chaplaincy

Spiritual support offered to patient, parents/family
with child who has a chronic illness and associated
concerns
Goals:

Spiritual support provided to patient,
parents/family
Referral to community spiritual resource(s) as
indicated

Social work

Assessment of emotional/social factors related to
illness

Financial resource information (e.g., needed supplies)
Referral(s) to identified community resources
Goals:
> Problem identification and referral(s) to resources

Discharge planning nurse/team

Evaluation
Problem identification
Referral to home care nurse to continue education in home and assist with insulin injection/home glucose monitoring until family unit is independent
Goals:
> Referral(s) to community health resources for follow-up

9. **Nursing goals and outcomes**

Daily implementation of care plan, created within _____ hours of admission and updated and/or reevaluated q _____ hours or as indicated by patient's condition
Return to self-care or status prior to hospitalization, with functional mobility and ambulation
Blood sugars maintained within normal range for patient
Infection-free, afebrile
Parent/other caregiver able to verbalize/demonstrate care regimens
Compliance demonstrated while an inpatient
Process of acceptance of chronic illness initiated, progressing
Areas of nutrition, exercise, insulin preparation, administration, and actions verbalized correctly prior to discharge
Signs, symptoms of hyperglycemia/hypoglycemia and actions taught
Child/caregiver able to effectively use home glucose monitoring system

10. **Potential discharge plans for this patient**
    Discharge to home, self-care
    Discharge to home with family able to meet care needs
    as taught and follow-up from physician
    Referral to community home nursing services

Diabetes Mellitus in Pregnancy

◆

1. **Assessment of the patient problem**

   Obtain subjective data from the patient, family, or caregiver(s)

2. **Associated nursing diagnoses**

   Activity intolerance
   Activity intolerance, high risk for
   Adjustment, impaired
   Anxiety
   Body image disturbance
   Body temperature, altered, high risk for
   Coping, ineffective family: compromised
   Coping, ineffective family: disabling
   Coping, ineffective individual
   Denial, ineffective
   Family processes, altered
   Fatigue
   Fear
   Fluid volume deficit, high risk for
   Fluid volume excess
   Gas exchange, impaired
   Grieving, anticipatory
   Grieving, dysfunctional
   Infection, high risk for
   Injury, high risk for
   Knowledge deficit (care of diabetes mellitus)
   Mobility, impaired physical
   Noncompliance (specify)
   Nutrition, altered: high risk for more than body requirements
   Nutrition, altered: less than body requirements
   Nutrition, altered: more than body requirements
   Pain
   Pain, chronic
   Parenting, altered

Sensory/perceptual alterations (specify) (visual,
auditory, kinesthetic, gustatory, tactile, olfactory)
Sexual dysfunction
Sexuality patterns, altered
Skin integrity, impaired
Skin integrity, impaired, high risk for
Spiritual distress (distress of the human spirit)
Thought processes, altered
Tissue integrity, impaired
Tissue perfusion, altered (specify type) (renal, cerebral,
cardiopulmonary, gastrointestinal, peripheral)

3. **Examples of objective data for documentation**

Vital signs
Level of consciousness
Tears, crying
Blood glucose levels
Urinary catheter presence
Lung sounds
Weight loss
Oxygen use
Intake and output
Skin color
Acetone presence
Frequent urination
Increased thirst
Excessive hunger
Nausea, vomiting
Fetal heart rate
Reactivity of nonstress test (NST)

4. **Examples of the assessment of the data**

Unstable vital signs (e.g., BP high or low, febrile,
change in vital signs)
Upset, depressed
IV infusing
Patent urinary catheter
Change in lung sounds
High blood pressure

Hyperglycemia
Hypoglycemia
Diabetic ketoacidosis
Nonstress test (NST) nonreactive, reactive

5. **Examples of potential medical problems for this patient**

Insulin shock
Urinary tract infection
Pneumonia or other process
Peripheral vascular disease
Leg or foot ulcers
Hyperglycemia
Hypoglycemia
Arterial occlusive disease
Cellulitis
Hypertension
Neuropathy
Retinopathy
Ketoacidosis (coma, death)
Vasculitis
Monilia or other infections
Local tissue atrophy
Nephropathy
Hydramnios
Premature rupture of membranes
Coma
Intrauterine fetal death
Pyelonephritis
Hydramnios
Other

6. **Examples of the documentation of potential nursing interventions/actions**

Assessed baseline knowledge regarding aspects of care related to diabetes mellitus
Vital signs being measured (specify routes) q _____
Evaluated level of consciousness
Emotional support provided to patient and family

Taught medication regimen

Support hose applied

Taught signs, symptoms of hyperglycemia/hypoglycemia

Taught patient to measure, record, and report blood sugars

Auscultation for respiratory baseline/changes performed

Foot care regimen implemented

Daily weights

Patient and caregiver taught to mix insulins

Observed for potential infection at wound site

Assessed for amount, site of fluid retention

Diet of _____ taught to patient and caregiver

Administered _____ units of _____ insulin sc

Taught patient and caregiver to draw up and administer insulin

Taught diabetes management regimens per facility protocol(s)

Taught patient/caregiver regarding diet and importance of eating at regular times

Blood glucose being monitored q _____ (call physician if over _____ or less than _____)

Taught survival skills/emergency measures to patient and family regarding hyperglycemia/hypoglycemia

Assessed and identified need for podiatry evaluation

Taught actions of ordered insulin(s)

Monitored pedal pulses

Taught safety measures regarding decreased sensation (e.g., to avoid heating pads)

Patient taught use of home glucose monitoring

Patient taught to count fetal movements

Taught relationship of exercise and diet

7. **Examples of the evaluations of the interventions/actions**

Blood glucose _____, within normal range for patient

Temperature rechecked at _____ PM; now _____, within normal range

Patient demonstrated correct procedure of _____
as taught
Observed no evidence of infection at site; no heat,
redness, swelling, drainage, or increased temperature
noted

8. **Other services that may be indicated and their associated interventions and goals/outcomes**

   Nurse aide
   Personal care
   ADL assistance
   Other duties
   Goals:
   > Effective personal care provided
   > Assist with ADLs
   > Patient clean and comfortable

   Chaplaincy
   Spiritual support offered to patient,
   family/caregiver(s)
   Goals:
   > Spiritual support provided to patient,
   > family/caregiver(s)

   Social work
   Assessment of social and emotional factors
   Counseling
   Financial assistance
   Goals:
   > Resources identified and referral(s) made to
   > community programs

   Discharge planning nurse/team
   Comprehensive evaluation of patient's needs
   Goals:
   > Patient and family ready for discharge
   > Community resources contacted
   > Home nursing care referral initiated

9. **Nursing goals and outcomes**

   Diabetes mellitus controlled as evidenced by blood
   glucose within normal range for patient
   Patient/family taught regarding insulin or other
   medications, diet regimens, and emergency measures
   Compliance demonstrated while a patient; able to care
   for infant
   Patient delivered a healthy infant

10. **Potential discharge plans for this patient**

   Discharge to home; goals achieved
   Patient understands her illness and demonstrates care
   taught regarding diabetes mellitus management
   Patient discharged postpartum; self-care and able to
   care for infant
   Patient discharged, still antepartal, with home nursing
   services follow-up

Newborn Care

◆

1. **Assessment of the patient problem**
   Obtain subjective data from family or caregiver(s)

2. **Associated nursing diagnoses**
   Airway clearance, ineffective
   Anxiety
   Breastfeeding, effective
   Breastfeeding, ineffective
   Comfort, alteration in
   Constipation
   Family processes, altered
   Fear
   Infection, high risk for
   Injury, high risk for
   Knowledge deficit (care of a newborn)
   Nutrition, altered: high risk for more than body
   requirements
   Nutrition, altered: less than body requirements
   Nutrition, altered: more than body requirements
   Parenting, altered
   Urinary elimination, altered patterns
   Skin integrity, impaired
   Thermoregulation, ineffective

3. **Examples of objective data for documentation**
   Findings from newborn assessment: height, weight,
   head circumference
   Cyanosis
   Apgar
   Rash
   Immediate lab data: glucose, pH, etc.
   Heart, respiratory rate
   Temperature
   Crying
   Sucking

Bottle-feeding
Feeding
Rh of infant
Umbilicus description
Skin mottling
Presence of eye discharge
Jaundice

4. **Examples of the assessment of the data**
   Infant breastfeeding
   Temperature remains _____
   Infant voiding
   Weight change of _____ lb (g)
   Irritable
   Infant positioned on right side after feeding
   Father remaining with mother and infant to assist in
   positioning
   Strong suck

5. **Examples of the potential medical problems for
   this patient**
   Respiratory distress syndrome
   Sepsis
   Low birth weight
   Birth injuries
   Prematurity
   Hyperbilirubinemia
   Blood incompatibilities
   Seizures
   Metabolic problems such as low blood sugar
   Other

6. **Examples of the documentation of potential
   nursing interventions/actions**
   Vital signs monitored on admission; being monitored
   q _____ per hospital policy
   Assessment of infant performed on admission to
   nursery

Infant brought to mother for breastfeeding on demand
schedule
Teaching about feeding, bathing regimen initiated
Physician contacted of change noted in infant
Weight obtained
Emotional support provided to new parents

7. **Examples of the evaluations of the
   interventions/actions**

   Infant sleeping after breastfeeding
   Infant retained feeding
   Parents verbalized comfort level with bathing
   procedures taught by RN
   Weight remains stable for infant

8. **Other services that may be indicated and their
   associated interventions and goals/outcomes**

   Nurse aide

   Personal care
   Goals:
       Effective personal care provided

   Chaplaincy

   Spiritual support offered to parents/caregiver(s)
   Goals:
       Spiritual support provided to parents/caregiver(s)

   Social work

   Assessment of identified problem(s)
   Counseling
   Financial assistance
       Goals:
       Resources identified and referral(s) made to
       community program

   Discharge planning nurse

   Evaluation of infant's and family's needs

Goals:
    Parents and infant ready for discharge
    Community resource referral(s) initiated (e.g.,
    home nursing service follow-up)

9. **Nursing goals and outcomes**
    Parents able to care for newborn
    Infant feeding and retaining nutrition
    Cord site clean, drying, without infection
    Temperature stable
    Adequate respiratory status

10. **Potential discharge plans for this patient**
    Discharge to home; goals achieved
    Family able to care for infant at home

Post–Cesarean Section Care

◆

1. **Assessment of the patient problem**
   Obtain subjective data from the patient, family, or
   caregiver(s)

2. **Associated nursing diagnoses**
   Anxiety
   Body image disturbance
   Breastfeeding, effective
   Breastfeeding, ineffective
   Constipation
   Coping, ineffective family: compromised
   Family processes, altered
   Fatigue
   Fear
   Growth and development, altered
   Infection, high risk for (e.g., urinary tract, uterus,
   wound site, breast, respiratory tract)
   Knowledge deficit (regarding self-care S/P C-section,
   infant care)
   Pain
   Parental role conflict
   Parenting, altered, high risk for
   Role performance, altered
   Sexual dysfunction
   Sexuality patterns, altered
   Skin integrity, impaired
   Sleep pattern disturbance
   Spiritual distress (distress of the human spirit)
   Urinary retention

3. **Examples of objective data for documentation**
   Vital signs
   Fundus description (firm, boggy, height)
   Lochia description
   Presence of urinary catheter

Prior C-section(s), date(s) where applicable
Tears, crying
Bowel sounds, movements
Presence of newborn, visitors
Intake and output
Presence of IV infusing and site description
Varicosities
Breath sounds
Alert, oriented x3
Breastfeeding
Positive Homan's sign
Incision site and type
Number of other children
History of problems with previous
pregnancies/deliveries
Number of live births/abortions
EDC; premature deliveries?
Birth control measures
Blood type and Rh

4. **Examples of the assessment of the data**
   Unable to sleep/rest
   New area of breast tenderness; mother has inverted
   nipples, cracked nipples, bleeding nipples
   Effective breastfeeding
   Mother able to rest with infant feeding schedule
   (specify)
   Patient voiding without pain or frequency after
   removal of catheter
   Patent urinary catheter
   Pain
   Weight loss or gain
   Fatigue
   Upset, crying
   Baby not feeding well

5. **Examples of potential medical problems for this patient**
   Anemia

Hemorrhoids
Uterine infection (endometritis)
Mastitis
Thrombophlebitis
Anesthesia complications
Hematomas
Urinary tract infection
Wound infection
Wound dehiscence
Uterine perforation
Pneumonia
Other complications of surgery
Bowel obstruction
Ileus
Pulmonary embolism
Amniotic fluid embolism
Other

6. **Examples of the documentation of potential nursing interventions/actions**

   Mother taught measures to relieve breast engorgement
   RN administered ordered analgesia of _____
   Teaching initiated regarding operative wound site care
   Fluids encouraged po; patient still has urinary catheter
   Infant brought to mother for breastfeeding on demand schedule
   Initial teaching begun regarding care of infant (see flow sheet)
   Physician contacted regarding patient's increased blood pressure
   Emotional support provided to new parents

7. **Examples of the evaluations of the interventions/actions**

   Patient verbalized relief of pain after ordered analgesia given
   Patient able to dress wound site as taught by RN
   Patient able to list signs, symptoms of wound infection/problem

Patient able to urinate without pain or frequency after catheter removal this AM

8. **Other services that may be indicated and their associated interventions and goals/outcomes**

   Nurse aide
   Personal care
   ADL assistance
   ROM of extremities if bedridden
   Infant care
   Goals:
   > Effective personal and infant care provided
   > Mother verbalizes that she feels clean and comfortable

   Chaplaincy
   Spiritual support offered to parents or caregiver(s)
   Goals:
   > Spiritual support provided to parents or caregiver(s)

   Social work
   Assessment of identified problem(s)
   Counseling
   Financial assistance
   Goals:
   > Resources identified and referral(s) made to community programs

   Discharge planning nurse/team
   Evaluation of new family needs
   Goals:
   > Parents and infant ready for discharge or other disposition
   > Community health referral(s) initiated for follow-up

9. **Nursing goals and outcomes**
   Daily implementation of care plan, created within

_____ hours of admission and updated and/or reevaluated q _____ hours or as indicated by patient's condition

Return to self-care or status prior to hospitalization, pain-free with functional mobility and ambulation

Parents able to demonstrate, verbalize care of newborn

Infection-free

Mother able to demonstrate wound site care

Effective feeding of newborn occurring

Pain controlled

Has had bowel movement; able to void without pain or frequency

10. Potential discharge plans for this patient

Discharge to home; self-care and able to care for infant

Discharge to home with follow-up support of home nursing services for identified problem(s) and birth control counseling where appropriate

Postpartal Care

◆

1. **Assessment of the patient problem**

   Obtain subjective data from the patient, family, or caregiver(s)

2. **Associated nursing diagnoses**

   Anxiety
   Body image disturbance
   Breastfeeding, effective
   Breastfeeding, ineffective
   Constipation
   Coping, ineffective family: compromised
   Family processes, altered
   Fatigue
   Fear
   Growth and development, altered
   Infection, high risk for
   Knowledge deficit (regarding care)
   Pain
   Role performance, altered
   Sexuality patterns, altered
   Sleep pattern disturbance
   Urinary retention

3. **Examples of objective data for documentation**

   Vital signs
   Weight
   Lochia
   Fundus height/consistency
   Varicosities
   Intake and output
   Breastfeeding
   Blood type and Rh
   Positive Homan's sign
   Urinary catheter
   Presence of infant or visitor(s)

Delivery date
Incision site and type (episiotomy and laceration)
Number of other children
Presence of hemorrhoids

4. **Examples of the assessment of the data**
   Unable to sleep
   New area of breast tenderness, redness, or heat
   Mother able to rest with infant feeding schedule
   (specify)
   Patient voiding without pain or frequency

5. **Examples of potential medical problems for this patient**
   Hemorrhage
   Hemorrhoids
   Uterine infection (endometritis)
   Mastitis
   Thrombophlebitis
   Anesthesia complications
   Hematomas
   Urinary tract infection
   Anemia
   Other

6. **Examples of the documentation of potential nursing interventions/actions**
   Mother taught measures to relieve breast engorgement
   RN notified obstetrician regarding patient's blood
   pressure
   Intake and output being monitored

7. **Examples of the evaluations of the interventions/actions**
   Pain relief verbalized after administration of ordered
   analgesia
   Breasts noted to be without redness, unusual
   engorgement

8. **Other services that may be indicated and their associated interventions and goals/outcomes**

   Nurse aide

   Personal care
   ADL assistance
   Other duties
   Goals:
   > Effective personal care provided
   > Patient clean and comfortable

   Chaplaincy

   Spiritual support offered to patient,
   family/caregiver(s)
   Goals:
   > Spiritual support provided to patient,
   > family/caregiver(s)
   > Referral to community spiritual resource(s) as
   > indicated

   Social work

   Assessment of emotional/social factors impacting on
   health
   Financial assistance
   Goals:
   > Referred to identified community resources

   Discharge planning nurse/team

   Evaluation of needs following discharge
   Goals:
   > Patient referred to home nursing program for
   > follow-up per physician order(s)
   > Patient notified of plan prior to discharge

9. **Nursing goals and outcomes**

   Parents able to demonstrate, verbalize care of newborn
   Mother able to care for self postpartum

10. **Potential discharge plans for this patient**

Discharge to home; self-care and able to care for infant

Discharge to home with follow-up support of home nursing services for identified problem

Patient to return to physician for follow-up and birth control counseling where appropriate

Sickle Cell Anemia (Care of the Child with)

◆

1. **Assessment of the patient problem**
   Obtain subjective data from the patient, parents, or caregiver(s)

2. **Associated nursing diagnoses**
   Body image disturbance
   Coping, ineffective family: compromised
   Coping, ineffective family: disabling
   Family processes, altered
   Fatigue
   Fear
   Fluid volume deficit
   Fluid volume deficit, high risk for
   Grieving, anticipatory
   Growth and development, altered
   Infection, high risk for
   Injury, high risk for
   Mobility, impaired physical
   Nutrition altered: less than body requirements
   Pain
   Pain, chronic
   Skin integrity, impaired
   Skin integrity, impaired, high risk for
   Tissue perfusion, altered (specify type) (renal cerebral, cardiopulmonary, gastrointestinal, peripheral)
   Sexual dysfunction

3. **Examples of objective data for documentation**
   Vital signs
   Swelling
   Use of oxygen
   Results of blood tests (e.g., WBC, HCT, HGB)
   Weight

Cough, chills
Jaundiced sclera
Date(s) of last hospitalization
Pain _____ (location)
Shortness of breath
Crying/tears
Irritability

4. **Examples of the assessment of the data**
   Acute crisis
   Severe pain
   Febrile
   Dehydration
   IV patent and infusing at ordered rate of _____
   Abdominal (or other location of) pain
   Patient needs analgesia for pain relief
   Positive blood cultures
   Productive cough
   Enlarged spleen

5. **Examples of potential medical problems for this patient**
   Infections/sepsis
   Congestive heart failure
   Renal failure
   Respiratory distress/pneumonia
   Delayed growth and sexual maturation
   Osteomyelitis
   Retinopathy
   Priapism
   Splenomegaly
   Involvement of any major organ
   Complications of blood transfusion
   CVA
   Delayed growth and sexual maturation
   Other

6. **Examples of the documentation of the potential nursing intervention/actions**

   Comprehensive nursing evaluation of all systems completed

   Pain assessment performed, including site(s), frequency, character, and history of obtaining relief

   Measures taken to achieve pain control as quickly as possible

   Emotional support provided to child and family/caregiver(s)

   Family/patient taught importance of adequate hydration/nutritional status

   Assessment completed of site(s), amount of swelling

   Patient repositioned for comfort

   Administered ordered analgesic

   Care to stasis ulcers performed per protocol

   Venipunctures obtained as ordered

   Vital signs being monitored q hour as ordered

   Daily weights

   Intake and output being monitored

   Auscultation of breath sounds completed

   ROM exercises completed

7. **Examples of the evaluations of the interventions/actions**

   IV patent and site without redness, tenderness, swelling, or other signs of infection/infiltration

   Temperature rechecked; now _____, within normal range for patient

   Site(s) without exudate, warmth, or tenderness

   Pain controlled as evidenced by pain now at _____ on scale of 1 to 10

   Parent/caregiver demonstrated correct procedure of ROM as taught by RN

   Paient maintaining ordered complete bed rest

Pain relief verbalized after RN administered ordered analgesic

Decreased swelling noted in affected knee; had increased ROM

Abdomen no longer distended

Lab value now _____, within normal range for patient

Positive response to new medication; patient verbalizes feels better, is eating again

Patient tolerated transfusion of packed red blood cells with no adverse effects

Urinary output normal for patient's age

Patient and parent able to rest between planned interventions

Patient's intake has improved as evidenced by

_____

Weight gain of _____, up from weight of (date and weight)

Negative blood cultures

Lungs, breath sounds clear on auscultation

Affected joint now without warmth, swelling, or pain

Patient no longer experiencing shortness of breath

8. **Other services that may be indicated and their associated interventions/actions**

Nurse aide

Personal care

ADL assistance

Other duties

Goals:

> Effective personal care provided
> Patient clean and comfortable

Occupational therapy

Evaluation

Conservation-of-energy techniques

Teach safe use of assistive devices

ADL retraining

Goals:

> Increased functional mobility; self-care in ADL; using conservation-of-energy techniques

Chaplaincy
  Spiritual support offered to
  patient/family/caregiver(s)
Goals:
  Spiritual support provided to patient,
  family/caregiver(s)
  Referral to community spiritual resource(s) as
  indicated

Social work
Assessment of emotional/social factors impacting on
health
Financial resource information to parents/caregiver(s)
Referral(s) to community resources
Goals:
  Problem identification and referral(s) to resources
  Meeting with patient, family prior to discharge to
  communicate plan
  Referral to community support group

Discharge planning nurse/team
Comprehensive patient/family evaluation
Communication of identified needs to team
Referral(s) as indicated based on needs assessment
Goals:
  Evaluation for and referral(s) to identified
  community programs

9. **Nursing Goals and Outcomes**
    Daily implementation of care plan, created within
    _____ hours of admission and updated and/or
    reevaluated q _____ hours or as indicated by patient's
    condition
    Return to self-care or status prior to hospitalization,
    pain-free with functional mobility and ambulation
    Pain controlled
    Hydration/nutritional status adequate
    Infection-free
    Parents/caregiver(s) able to care for patient
    Parents/caregiver(s) can identify precipitating factors
    to be avoided

10. Potential discharge plans for this patient

Discharge to home, self-care
Discharge to home with parents/caregiver(s) able to care for patient
Discharge to home with home nursing care follow-up
Symptom-controlled death in hospital

Surgical Care of the Child

◆

1. **Assessment of the patient problem**

   Obtain subjective data from the patient, parents, or
   caregiver(s)

2. **Associated nursing diagnoses**

   Activity intolerance
   Activity intolerance, high risk for
   Adjustment, impaired
   Airway clearance, ineffective
   Anxiety
   Breathing pattern, ineffective
   Constipation
   Coping, family: potential for growth
   Family processes, altered
   Fatigue
   Fear
   Fluid volume deficit, high risk for
   Fluid volume excess
   Gas exchange, impaired
   Growth and development, altered
   Infection, high risk for
   Injury, high risk for
   Nutrition altered: less than body requirements
   Oral mucous membrane, altered
   Pain
   Pain, chronic
   Parental role conflict
   Parenting, altered
   Parenting, altered, high risk for
   Self-care deficit, bathing/hygiene
   Self-care deficit, dressing/grooming
   Self-care deficit, feeding
   Self-care deficit, toileting
   Sensory/perceptual alterations (specify) (visual,
   auditory, kinesthetic, gustatory, tactile, olfactory)

Sexuality patterns, altered
Skin integrity, impaired
Skin integrity, impaired, high risk for
Sleep pattern disturbance
Social interaction, impaired
Spiritual distress (distress of the human spirit)
Urinary elimination, altered patterns

3. **Examples of objective data for documentation**
   Weight(s)
   Vital signs
   Bleeding
   Time of last meal
   Use of glasses
   Presence of parents, other visitors
   Absence of parents, other visitors
   Signed consent
   Vomiting
   Lab or other diagnostic tests
   Dressing(s)
   Intake and output
   Abdominal distention
   Crying, tears
   Hypotonic bowel sounds

4. **Examples of the assessment of the data**
   Unstable vital signs (specify)
   Acute abdominal (or other site) pain
   Weight loss
   Patent urinary catheter
   Febrile
   Ileus
   Parent tearful after meeting with physician regarding
   test results
   Pain

5. **Examples of potential medical problems for this patient**

Those complications specific to the surgical procedure
Wound infection
Pneumonia
Atelectasis
Fluid volume overload
Urinary tract infection
Other infections
Dehydration
Electrolyte imbalances
Wound dehiscence
Constipation
Other

6. **Examples of the documentation of potential nursing interventions/actions**

Comprehensive baseline nursing assessment completed during admission
RN explained what will occur to child with parents in attendance
Teaching child about dressing site and IV initiated; child demonstrated understanding by bandaging doll in same site
Emotional support provided to child and parents
RN checked for presence of signed informed consent on chart
Patient prepped; site cleansed per physician order(s)
Child transported to OR with pajama bottoms on, child's blanket, stuffed toy
OR nurse confirmed that parents will stay with child during induction procedure
Postoperative assessment of child performed on return to unit
Vital signs being measured q _____ on unit postoperatively

Medication of _____ administered for pain as ordered

RN reevaluated postoperative wound site and dressings

Intake and output being measured q _____

Patient turned and repositioned by RN

Encouraged patient to deep breathe and cough

Parents taught importance of turning/movement, deep breathing and coughing, assisting RN

Physician notified of change in condition

Assessment of child's hydration/nutritional status performed by RN

Child noted to have first bowel movement postoperatively; e.g., small, soft at _____ PM

Postoperative assessment of pain performed (amount, character, relief measures)

Child assisted with blow bottles or incentive spirometer q _____

Child reoriented by parents on awakening on pediatric unit

Child being offered favorite fluids as recommended by parents

IV antibiotic of _____ hung at _____ AM per physician order(s)

Physician notified of abdominal distention

7. **Examples of the evaluations of the interventions/actions**

Child able to play and then sleep after administration of analgesic

Lab value of _____, within normal range for patient

Physician notified of change identified of _____

Mother/father demonstrated correct procedure of _____ as taught by RN

Temperature rechecked at _____ PM, after antipyretic; now _____

Weight decreased to _____ lb

Patient out in playroom with parent

Patient now eating, since foods of choice put on trays

8. **Other services that may be indicated and their associated interventions and goals/outcomes**

   Nurse aide
   Personal care
   ADL assistance
   Other duties
   Goals:
   > Effective personal care provided
   > Patient clean and comfortable

   Chaplaincy
   > Spiritual support offered to child,
   > parents/caregiver(s)
   Goals:
   > Spiritual support provided to child,
   > parents/caregiver(s)

   Social work
   Assessment of factors impacting on health
   Financial resource information to parents/caregiver(s)
   Referral(s) to community resources
   Goals:
   > Problem identification and referral(s) to identified
   > resources
   > Meeting with child, parents prior to discharge to
   > communicate plan

   Discharge planning nurse/team
   Patient/family evaluation
   Referral(s) to community health resources
   Goals:
   > Appropriate referral(s) to identified community
   > resources

   Home care nurse
   Wound care, dressing changes

9. **Nursing goals and outcomes**

Daily implementation of care plan, created within
_____ hours of admission and updated and/or
reevaluated q _____ hours or as indicated by patient's
condition
Return to self-care or status prior to hospitalization,
pain-free with functional mobility and ambulation
Surgical site healing without pain, infection
Child able to resume play, mobility
Adequate hydration/nutritional status
Child's diet has resumed
Child able to void; has bowel movements
Parents/caregiver(s) able to care for child

10. **Potential discharge plans for this patient**

Discharge to home; parents providing care for child
Discharge to home with follow-up by community
home nursing services

Appendix A

NANDA-Approved Nursing Diagnoses

Activity intolerance
Activity intolerance, high risk for
Adjustment, impaired
Airway clearance, ineffective
Anxiety
Aspiration, high risk for
Body image disturbance
Body temperature, altered, high risk for
Bowel incontinence
Breastfeeding, effective
Breastfeeding, ineffective
Breathing pattern, ineffective
Cardiac output, decreased
Communication, impaired verbal
Constipation
Constipation, colonic
Constipation, perceived
Coping, defensive
Coping, family: potential for growth
Coping, ineffective family: compromised
Coping, ineffective family: disabling
Coping, ineffective individual
Decisional conflict (specify)
Denial, ineffective
Diarrhea
Disuse syndrome, high risk for
Diversional activity deficit
Dysreflexia

Family processes, altered
Fatigue
Fear
Fluid volume deficit (1)
Fluid volume deficit (2)
Fluid volume deficit, high risk for
Fluid volume excess
Gas exchange, impaired
Grieving, anticipatory
Grieving, dysfunctional
Growth and development, altered
Health maintenance, altered
Health-seeking behaviors (specify)
Home maintenance management, impaired
Hopelessness
Hyperthermia
Hypothermia
Incontinence, functional
Incontinence, reflex
Incontinence, stress
Incontinence, total
Incontinence, urge
Infection, high risk for
Injury, high risk for
Knowledge deficit (specify)
Mobility, impaired physical
Noncompliance (specify)
Nutrition, altered: high risk for more than body
   requirements
Nutrition, altered: less than body requirements
Nutrition, altered: more than body requirements
Oral mucous membrane, altered
Pain
Pain, chronic
Parental role conflict
Parenting, altered

Parenting, altered, high risk for
Personal identity disturbance
Poisoning, high risk for
Post-trauma response
Powerlessness
Protection, altered
Rape-trauma syndrome
Rape-trauma syndrome; compound reaction
Rape-trauma syndrome: silent reaction
Role performance, altered
Self-care deficit, bathing/hygiene
Self-care deficit, dressing/grooming
Self-care deficit, feeding
Self-care deficit, toileting
Self-esteem disturbance
Self-esteem, chronic low
Self-esteem, situational low
Sensory/perceptual alterations (specify) (visual,
   auditory, kinesthetic, gustatory, tactile, olfactory)
Sexual dysfunction
Sexuality patterns, altered
Skin integrity, impaired
Skin integrity, impaired, high risk for
Sleep pattern disturbance
Social interaction, impaired
Social isolation
Spiritual distress (distress of the human spirit)
Suffocation, high risk for
Swallowing, impaired
Thermoregulation, ineffective
Thought processes, altered
Tissue integrity, impaired
Tissue perfusion, altered (specify type) (renal,
   cerebral, cardiopulmonary, gastrointestinal,
   peripheral)
Trauma, high risk for

Unilateral neglect
Urinary elimination, altered patterns
Urinary retention
Violence, high risk for: self-directed or directed at
  others

Appendix B

Services Provided by Other Disciplines

PHYSICAL THERAPY

Physical therapy (PT) involves initial patient evaluation, the development of an appropriate plan of care, skilled teaching, and the development of maintenance exercise programs for individuals who have physical injuries, disabilities, or are postsurgical and have lost normal physical functioning. Physical therapists often use physical modalities such as heat, light, electricity, cold, joint mobilization, postural drainage/breathing exercises, and other therapeutic exercises to increase normal physical functioning for such patients. Physical therapists are also experts in gait evaluation, as well as gait training and treatment for conditions involving (but not limited to) deficits in neurological, skeletal, muscular, integumentary, and respiratory systems. Also, physical therapists have become increasingly involved in the physical rehabilitation of patients suffering from cardio-vascular pathologies.

OCCUPATIONAL THERAPY

Occupational therapy (OT) evaluation and treatment may involve any of the following areas: muscle strength, fine motor coordination, joint range of motion (ROM), perceptual motor skills, sensory testing, communication skills, daily life skills (including activities of daily living [ADL], home management, and reality orientation). Treatment modalities may also include splints, slings, and other adaptive equipment such as self-help devices, and specially designed clothing.

OT treatment is focused on teaching compensation for limitations in function that result from disease or disability. Goals of treatment change as the patient improves or loses function as a result of a debilitating disease process. OT treatment goals are individualized to the patient's specific needs at any given time and are reevaluated on an ongoing basis.

SPEECH-LANGUAGE PATHOLOGY SERVICES

Speech-language pathology (SLP) services are vital rehabilitative services indicated for patients with varied speech and/or swallowing disorders. Other areas include voice skills, language, speech formulation, breath control, pacing, swallowing, and reading comprehension.

Often it is the nurse who is in a position to identify the need for SLP services in the admission assessment and ongoing evaluations. Two areas the nurse should routinely consider are the potential need for a hearing evaluation and the probability of swallowing disorders in the patient with a cerebrovascular accident (CVA).

CHAPLAINCY SERVICES

The hospital chaplain ministers to a population that spans the continuum from birth through death. The chaplain, like the nurse, interfaces with patients and their families at some of the most difficult times of their lives. This struggle with the meaning of life, experienced by all who are hospitalized, is the work of the chaplain. The chaplain counsels regardless of any formal "religious" beliefs.

The role varies, based on patient, family, or staff

needs, and may include bereavement counseling, serving on the hospital ethics committee, or performing the sacrament of the sick. Nursing staff may also be involved in scheduled worship services for staff, visitors, and patients. The chaplain facilitates the patient's movement toward his or her own resolution of life's questions.

Other services may include baptism, blessings or prayers with patients and family members, or hospice staff support. Patients who may benefit from chaplaincy services include those for whom the nursing diagnosis "spiritual distress (distress of the human spirit)" has been identified by the nursing staff.

SOCIAL WORK SERVICES

Social work involves identification, treatment, and patient support for social, emotional, and environmental problems associated with an illness or disability. Medical social workers (MSWs) assist patients and their families with problem solving, serve as patient advocates, and help patients take advantage of resources that may be available to them. They may also provide counseling to patients and their families.

PERSONAL EMERGENCY RESPONSE SYSTEMS

Personal emergency response systems (PERS) are a unique form of technology that links the frail or elderly with community resources, neighbors, or a friend at the push of a button. Although there are different brands of PERS, all brands are telephone service dependent. PERS may be appropriate for patients returning home alone after surgery or for patients who live alone and are at risk for falls. All

PERS signal for help at the push of a button, which must be worn by the PERS "subscriber" at all times for the system to be effective. Many hospitals offer this service on discharge, but the nurse is in a position to identify this need so that the referral is initiated.

HOSPICE CARE

Hospice care is sometimes appropriate for patients with an illness of a terminal nature. Hospice care focuses on comfort and quality of life to assist the patient and family in making every remaining day the best that it can be. Hospice is a philosophy and, as such, can be enacted in any setting, such as the home or an inpatient hospice unit. Palliative care, emotional support, and control of pain and other symptoms are some of the areas addressed by the hospice team. At team meetings the physician, the spiritual counselor, the primary nurse, the hospice volunteers, the social worker, and others assist the patient and family in meeting their unique needs.

After death, bereavement support services provided to the family are a key component of continued hospice care.

Appendix C

Abbreviations

aa	of each
A/B	acid-base ratio
ABD	abdomen
ac	ante cibum (before meals)
ACTH	adrenocorticotropic hormone
ad lib	as desired
ADL	activities of daily living
Adm	admission
ADR	adverse drug reaction
Amb	ambulatory
AMI	acute myocardial infarction
AR	apical rate
ARD	acute respiratory distress
as tol	as tolerated
ASD	atrial septal defect
AV	atrioventricular;arteriovenous
bid	bis in die (twice a day)
BP	blood pressure
BR	bed rest
BRP	bathroom privileges
BS	blood sugar
BUN	blood urea nitrogen
C	centigrade (°C)
CA	cancer; cardiac arrest

Cath	catheter
CBC	complete blood count
cc	cubic centimeter
CCU	coronary care unit
cg	centigram
CHD	congenital heart disease; coronary heart disease; congestive heart disease
CHF	congestive heart failure
cm	centimeter
CNS	central nervous system
COPD	chronic obstructive pulmonary disease
CPR	cardiopulmonary resuscitation
CSF	cerebrospinal fluid
CVA	cerebrovascular accident; costovertebral angle
CVP	central venous pressure
D & C	dilatation and curettage
dim	diminutive
DM	diabetes mellitus
DOE	dyspnea on exertion
D & S	dilatation and suction
D5W	dextrose 5% in water
Dx	diagnosis
ECG	electrocardiogram
Ecoli	*Escherichia coli*
ED	emergency department
EEG	electroencephalogram
EKG	electrocardiogram

EMG	electromyogram
ENT	ear, nose, and throat
ER	emergency room
FBS	fasting blood sugar
fx	fracture
g	gram
GI	gastrointestinal
GU	genitourinary
Hct	hematocrit
Hgb	hemoglobin
HHA	home health agency
HO	house officer
HOB	head of the bed
hs	hour of sleep
Hx	history
hypo	hypodermically
ICU	intensive care unit
IDDM	insulin-dependent diabetes mellitus
IM	intramuscular
I & O	intake and output
IPPB	intermittent positive-pressure breathing
LLE	lower left extremity
mEq	milliequivalent
MI	myocardial infarction
ml	milliliter
mm	millimeter
Mn	midnight
MSW	medical social worker

NA	nurse aide
nb	nota bene (note well)
NG or ng	nasogastric
NHP	nursing home placement
NIDDM	non-insulin-dependent diabetes mellitus
NPO	null per os (nothing by mouth)
O$_2$	oxygen
OD	right eye (oculus dexter)
OOB	out of bed
OR	operating room
os	mouth
OS	left eye (oculus sinister)
OT	occupational therapy
OU	both eyes (oculus uterique)
oz	ounces
P	pulse
pc	post cibum (after food; after meals)
PDR	*Physicians' Desk Reference*
PEEP	positive end-expiratory pressure
PERRLA	pupils equal, round, and reactive to light and accommodation
PKU	phenylketonuria
po	per os (by mouth)
prn	pro re nata (as needed; as desired)
PT	physical therapy
qam	every morning
qd	quaque die (every day)

qh	quaque hora (every hour)
q 2 h	every 2 hours
qid	quater in die (four times a day)
qod	quisque alius dies (every other day)
qs	quantum sufficiat (a sufficient quantity)
R	respiration
RBC	red blood cell, red blood count
RDS	respiratory distress syndrome
RLE	right lower extremity
ROM	range of motion
Rx	recipe (take/prescription)
sc	sub cutis (subcutaneously)
SLP	speech-language pathology
SOAP	subjective, objective, assessment plan
SOB	shortness of breath
SOS	si opus sit (if necessary)
S/P	status post
SR	sedimentation rate
stat	statim (immediately)
sub I	sublingual (under the tongue)
T	temperature
T & A	tonsillectomy and adenoidectomy
TIA	transient ischemic attack
tid	ter in die (3 times a day)
UA/C & B	urinalysis/culture and sensitivity

ung	ointment
URI	upper respiratory infection
UTI	urinary tract infection
vol %	volume percent
VS	vital signs (T, P, R, and BP)
WBC	white blood cell, white blood count
WIC	women, infants, and children program

BIBLIOGRAPHY

♦

Barker E: Brain tumor, frightening diagnosis, nursing challenge, *RN*, September 1990.

Bavin R: Documentation in pediatric critical care: more time at the bedside, *Pediatr Nurs*, p 387, September-October 1988.

Bergerson SR: Charting with a jury in mind, *Nursing 88*, p 51, April 1988.

Bobak I, Jensen M, Zalar M: *Essentials of maternity nursing*, ed 4, St Louis, 1989, Mosby–Year Book.

Boland M, Czarniecki L: Starting life with HIV, *RN*, January 1991.

Bradford EW: Preventing malpractice suits: what you can do, *Nursing 88*, p 63, September 1988.

Burke L, Murphy J: *Charting by exception: a cost-effective approach*, Albany, NY, 1988, Delmar.

Calfee BE: Are you restraining your patient's rights? *Nursing 88*, p 149, May 1988.

Carter K: Computer technology advances will help hospitals to compete, *Mod Healthc*, p 90, November 22.

Caruthers DD: Infectious pneumonia in the elderly, *Am J Nurs*, February 1990.

Clausen C: Staff RN: a discharge planner for every patient, *Nurs Manage*, p 58, November 1984.

Cline A: Streamlined documentation through exceptional charting, *Nurs Manage*, p 62, February 1989.

Collins HL: Legal risks of computer charting, *RN*, May 1990.

Creighton H: Legal significance of charting, part I, p 17, *Nurs Manage*, September 1987.

Cushing M: Hazards of the infiltrated IV, *Am J Nurs*, September 1990.

Cushing M: Law and orders, *Am J Nurs*, May 1990.

Cushing M: Listen and use your knowledge of science, *Am J Nurs*, November 1989.

Cuzzell JZ: Clues: itching and burning in skin folds, *Am J Nurs*, January 1990.

DeVita VT, editor: *AIDS: etiology, diagnosis, treatment and prevention*, Philadelphia, 1988, JB Lippincott.

Dibble SL, Savedra MC: Cystic fibrosis in adolescence: a new challenge, *Pediatr Nurs*, p 299, July-August 1988.

Dickinson R: Our way, VI ulcers heal, *RN*, July 1990.

Dossey B et al: *Holistic nursing: a handbook for practice*, Rockville, Md, 1988, Aspen.

Eggland ET: Charting: how and why to document your care daily—and fully, *Nursing 88*, p 76, November 1988.

Febry D, Nash D: Hypertension: the nurse's role, *RN*, November 1990.

Ferguson GH, Hildman T, Nichols B: The effect of nursing care planning systems on patient outcomes, *J Nurs Adm*, p 30, September 1987.

Ferri FF: *Practical guide to the care of the medical patient*, ed 2, St Louis, 1987, Mosby–Year Book.

Feutz SA: Legal implications of institutional standards for nurses, *J Nurs Adm*, p 4, July-August 1989.

Fiesta J: Look beyond your state for your standards of care, *Nursing 86*, p 41, August 1986.

Fisher CW: Legally speaking: the abnormal infant, protecting yourself against blame, *RN*, April 1990.

Fox-Ungar E, Guilbault K: Documentation: communicating professionalism, *Nurs Manage*, p 65, January 1989.

George MR: Cystic fibrosis: not just a pediatric problem anymore, *RN*, September 1990.

Glondys BA: *Today's challenge: content of the health record; documentation requirements in the medical record*, ed 2, Chicago, 1988, American Medical Record Association.

Greene E: Clues to a code, *RN*, July 1990.

Gropper EI: Does your charting reflect your worth?" *Geriatr Nurs*, p 99, March-April 1988.

Guido GW: *Legal issues in nursing: a source book for practice*, Norwalk, Conn, 1988, Appleton & Lange.

Harvey BL: Your patient's discharge plan: does it include home-care referral? *Nursing 81*, p 48, July 1981.

Heater BS et al: Helping patients recover faster, *Am J Nurs*, October 1990.

Herrick KM, McCullough S: Introducing nurses to computers in a multi-hospital environment, *Nurs Manage*, p 31, July 1989.

Hopkins JL, editor: Keeping the record straight: guidelines for charting, *QRC Advisor*, p 7, January 1990.

Iyer PW: New trends in charting, *Nursing 91*, p 48, January 1991.

Janson-Bjerklie S: Status asthmaticus, *Am J Nurs*, p 52, September 1990.

Kim MJ, McFarland GK, McLane AM: *Pocket guide to nursing diagnoses*, ed 4, St Louis, 1990, Mosby–Year Book.

Lampe S: Focus charting: a patient centered approach, *Creative Nurs Manage*, 1988.

Lenkman S: Management information systems and the role of the nurse vendor, *Nurs Clin North Am*, p 557, September 1985.

Luquire R: Six common causes of nursing liability, *Nursing 88*, p 61, November 1988.

McArthur J: AIDS dementia, *RN*, March 1990.

McCaffery M: Nurses lead the way to new priorities, *Am J Nurs*, October 1990.

McElroy D, Herbelin K: Writing a better patient care plan, *Nursing 88*, p 50, February 1988.

McEntyre R: *Practical guide to the care of the surgical patient*, St Louis, 1989, Mosby–Year Book.

Mehmert PA, Dickel CA, McKeighen RJ: Computerizing nursing diagnosis, *Nurs Manage*, p 24, July 1989.

Murphy J, Beglinger JE, Johnson B: Charting by exception: meeting the challenge of cost containment, *Nurs Manage*, p 56, February 1988.

Murphy J, Burke LJ: Charting by exception: a more efficient way to document, *Nursing 90*, May 1990.

Naccavato M, Kresevic D: Caring for adults who have cystic fibrosis, *Am J Nurs*, November 1989.

Neubauer MP: Legally speaking: careful charting—your best defense, *RN*, p 77, November 1990.

Novak LT: Accelerated recovery technique: a new approach to abdominal surgery, *Nursing 90*, November 1990.

Nursing 81 Books, Nursing Skillbook Series: *Documenting patient care responsibly*, Horsham, Pa, 1980, Intermed Communications.

Olson EV: Hazards of immobility, *Am J Nurs*, March 1990.

Philcher M: Post-discharge care: how to follow up, *Nursing 86*, p 50, August 1986.

Philpott M: Twenty good rules for good charting, *Nursing 86*, August 1986.

Rabinow J: Discharging patients: do you know all your legal risks? *Nurs Life*, p 26, March-April 1987.

Rivers R, Williamson N: Sickle cell anemia, complex disease, nursing challenge, *RN*, June 1990.

Rowland MA: Myths and facts about postop discomfort, *Am J Nurs*, May 1990.

Rust D, Kloppenborg E: Don't underestimate the lumpectomy patient's needs, *RN*, March 1990.

Rutkowksi B: How D.R.G.s are changing your charting, *Nursing 85*, p 49, October 1985.

Sande M, Volberding A: *The medical management of AIDS*, Philadelphia, 1990, WB Saunders.

Taravella S: Denver AIDS-care center catches on as model, *Mod Healthc*, p 45, November 1989.

Vandenbosch TM: How to use a pain flow sheet effectively, *Nursing 88*, p 50, August 1988.

Wake MM: Nursing care delivery systems, *J Nurs Adm*, p 47, May 1990.

Weeks LC, Darrah P: The documentation dilemma: a practical solution, *J Nurs Adm*, p 22, November 1985.

Whaley LF, Wong DL: *Essentials of pediatric nursing*, ed 3, St Louis, 1989, Mosby–Year Book.

INDEX

◆

DATE DUE

GAYLORD   PRINTED IN U.S.A.